100 Questions & Answers About Your Child's Cancer

William L. Carroll, MD

Stephen D. Hassenfeld Children's Center
for Cancer and Blood Disorders
NYU Medical Center and
Mount Sinai Medical Center

Jessica B. Reisman, CSW

Stephen D. Hassenfeld Children's Center
for Cancer and Blood Disorders
NYU Medical Center

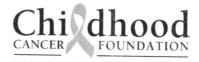

Chi dhood
CANCER FOUNDATION
CANDLELIGHTERS CANADA

This book is provided to you by the Childhood Cancer Foundation – Candlelighters Canada. We are a national, volunteer governed, charitable organization dedicated to improving the quality of life for children with cancer and their families. We will achieve our mission through undertaking and supporting national initiatives resulting in the increased survival and wellbeing of our children, and ultimately a cure for all childhood cancers. WE WILL WIN!

www.childhoodcancer.ca   Toll free #: 1800-363-1062

Sudbury, Massachusetts

BOSTON   TORONTO   LONDON   SINGAPORE

World Headquarters
Jones and Bartlett
Publishers
40 Tall Pine Drive
Sudbury, MA 01776
info@jbpub.com
www.jbpub.com

Jones and Bartlett
Publishers Canada
2406 Nikanna Road
Mississauga, ON L5C 2W6
CANADA

Jones and Bartlett
Publishers International
Barb House, Barb Mews
London W6 7PA
UK

Library of Congress Cataloging-in-Publication Data

Carroll, William L.
  100 questions & answers about your child's cancer / William L. Carroll. -- 1st ed.
    p. cm.
  Includes index.
  ISBN 0-7637-3140-4 (pbk.)
    1. Cancer in children--Popular works. 2. Cancer in children--Miscellanea.   I. Title.
II. Title: One hundred questions and answers about your child's cancer.
RC281.C4C424 2004
618.92'994--dc22

                                                                2004014814

Production Credits
Chief Executive Officer: Clayton Jones
Chief Operating Officer: Don W. Jones, Jr.
Executive V.P. & Publisher: Robert W. Holland, Jr.
V.P., Sales and Marketing: William J. Kane
V.P., Design and Production: Anne Spencer
V.P., Manufacturing and Inventory Control: Therese Bräuer
Executive Publisher: Christopher Davis
Special Projects Editor: Elizabeth Platt
Editorial Assistant: Kathy Richardson
Senior Marketing Manager: Alisha Weisman
Marketing Associate: Matthew Payne
Cover Design: Philip Regan
Cover Image: © Andersen Ross/Getty Images
Printing and Binding: Malloy, Inc.
Cover Printing: Malloy, Inc.

Printed in the United States of America

08 07 06 05 04   10 9 8 7 6 5 4 3 2 1

Contents

When I was asked by Jessica Reisman and William Carroll to write the Foreword to *100 Questions & Answers About Your Child's Cancer*, I was not only honored by the invitation but also pleased to have the opportunity to preview a much needed resource for families faced with what might arguably be the worst possible news any parent can receive: their child has been diagnosed with cancer. Few other situations are accompanied by such shock, pain, stress, and terror stemming from fear of the unknown, complicated by a loss of control and too many questions that require immediate answers.

No matter how extensive the exchange of information between a provider and a family during a diagnostic conference, little in the way of information is retained or sometimes even effectively communicated given the emotionally charged nature of such an exchange. Repeating previously communicated facts, figures, explanations, signs, symptoms, treatment plans, and potential outcomes is always a necessity. I have always advised parents to ask as many questions and to ask the same question as many times as they feel necessary to understand. Dr. Carroll and Ms. Reisman in *100 Questions & Answers About Your Child's Cancer* provide an amazing resource to parents and other family members in their immediate period of greatest need and present information in an honest, organized, and compassionate manner. They prioritize those areas of notable concern for patients and families: cancer causes, the similarity between childhood cancer and adult cancers, the immediate need to know what they did or didn't do to cause their child's cancer or what they could have done to prevent it, and the risk of cancer in their other children.

Fortunately, the field of pediatric oncology has experienced some extraordinary successes. A half century ago a child with cancer nearly always had a fatal outcome. Today, more than 78% of all children with cancer can expect to be cured. This does not, unfortunately, mean that all childhood cancer patients have a nearly 80% chance of cure. Certain cancer types are still associated with cure rates which are far less than half that. In addition to the extraordinary success during this half century, clinicians have gained considerable insights into the biology of cancer, a result of which has been better understanding of molecular and genetic aberrations associated with the cause of specific tumors, as well as the potential for the identification of specific biologic targets to which new agents and drugs might be directed, so as to eliminate or curtail the growth of cancer cells selectively. Advances in technology have resulted in enhanced diagnostic imaging tools for staging as well as sophisticated laboratory evaluations for biologic classification systems which are used in predicting risk of treatment failure and optimizing therapy through the use of risk-adjusted treatment strategies.

Despite tremendous advances, clinical investigators have also learned to appreciate that the success must be tempered, since cures for childhood cancer come with a significant price in many cases due to the short-term and long-term side effects of the disease and its therapy, which unfortunately impact on quality of life. During the past decade, the recognition of potential adverse effects of therapy have resulted in nearly equal attention to reducing short-term and long-term toxicities as increasing chances for treatment success and cure in evaluating new therapy approaches.

The extraordinary improvements in outcome for children with cancer have only been possible because of the coordination of evidence-based medicine in improving cure standards at specialized pediatric cancer treatment centers. The evidence-basis for improved treatments have resulted from multi-center clinical trials, multi-discipline in nature, and coordinated by the pediatric cooperative clinical trials group, supported by the National Cancer Institute and now unified and collaborating together as the Children's Oncology Group. Essential to the success of previous and current trials is the participation of patients and families in treatment protocols which seek to either build upon past success and improve chances for a cure or decrease toxicities of therapy.

Unfortunately, despite tremendous improvements and the fact that nearly 80% of children with cancer will become long-term survivors cured of their disease, cancer remains the leading cause of death in children after the first year of age through adolescence. Each year in the United States, approximately 14,000 infants, children, adolescents, and young adults are diagnosed with cancer.

Childhood cancer impacts not only the patient but the entire family as well as friends, classmates, and playmates. Complications of childhood cancer extend beyond the physical, emotional, and behavioral for the affected child to include emotional, psychological, and financial for the family. A particularly appealing part of this book, in addition to Dr. Carroll and Ms. Reisman's ability to address many basic issues and concerns as well as generalizable details related to diagnosis, treatment planning, and delivery, is the section called Living and Coping with Cancer—which coincidentally has the largest number of questions and answers. Living and coping within the extended social dynamics of family, most especially for adolescents and young adults with the diagnosis of cancer, creates extraordinary challenges. The helpful advice imparted in this section, much of it in the form of shared personal experiences of similarly affected families, is poignant and credible—and it provides the assurance that some families have survived to share their own stories. Additional, more comprehensive diagnosis-specific information is available as well, at Internet sites provided by the American Society of Clinical Oncology, called People Living with Cancer (www.plwc.org). There is also a new and more comprehensive site for patients and families, a joint venture between the Children's Oncology Group and the National Childhood Cancer Foundation, called CureSearch (www.CureSearch.org) is scheduled for launch imminently.

I am confident that *100 Questions & Answers About Your Child's Cancer* will go a long way in providing much needed information to parents as well as reinforce information received from numerous sources. I'm certain that it will be a trustworthy companion to parents who may have never previously felt more isolated and alone. This is a must-read for all families facing what shouldn't have to be the most frightening experience of their life.

Gregory H. Reaman, M.D.
Chairman, Children's Oncology Group
Professor of Pediatrics
The George Washington University School of Medicine
and Health Sciences
August 16, 2004

The faces, the names, and the presentation change, but the reaction rarely differs: the looks of fear and sadness in the eyes and faces of parents (and caregivers) as they hear the shocking words, "Your child has cancer." Working in the field of pediatric hematology/oncology, we have witnessed this exchange countless times. Overwhelmed with shock, many parents admit that they retained very little of the initial information presented. As subsequent treatment ensues, parents struggle with unanswered questions.

Presented with limited time and resources, parents and caregivers would greatly benefit from a comprehensive resource. An accessible guide could provide them with a tool that they could review and learn from at their own pace, in their own way, on their terms. Our sincere hope is that this book serves as a resource to help provide some of the answers.

The field of pediatric oncology continues to grow with the onslaught of research and subsequent advancements. Ever-changing technology is increasing the chances for cure. With these advancements, there is a steadfast commitment to improving a patient's quality of life during and after treatment. The emphasis is not only on diagnosis and treatment, but also on "living and coping." A survivor is now defined as anyone who has received a diagnosis of cancer. This definition accurately identifies the courageous struggle every patient and family endures, regardless of outcome. The new, expanded focus also helps to ensure that patients and families living with cancer will be considered people first and a diagnosis second.

With this approach to pediatric cancer treatment, it is imperative that healthcare professionals work together to deliver all-inclusive care to their patients. A cancer diagnosis thrusts a family and patient into a new reality and forces them to depend on many different disciplines for support and guidance. Families can best be served when all aspects of care—psychosocial, medical, and emotional—are addressed. This book is an exciting example of a multi-disciplinary approach to cancer care.

We have had the honor and privilege of working with many exceptional patients and their families at NYU Medical Center/Hassenfeld Children's Center for Cancer and Blood Disorders. They have taught us countless lessons about the fragility and preciousness of life. Their honesty, courage, and determination, in the face of a life-threatening illness, has inspired us to write this book. The families have given us much more than we can ever return. This book is our humble attempt to give back. We hope that it serves as a valuable tool on the journey to health.

We would also like to acknowledge and thank our friends and colleagues at NYU Medical Center/ Hassenfeld Children's Center and Mount Sinai Medical Center. We greatly appreciate the valuable feedback and commentary that we received from patients, families, and staff. Their patience and assistance was invaluable and helped to make this book complete. Among them are Christy O'Keefe, MA, CCLS, Kelly Cervone, RN, CPNP, Lauren Fennimore, RN, CPNP, Dr. Eduvigis Cruz-Arrieta, Jackie Schmelkin, CSW, Lisa Montalto, RN, CPNP, Diane Rosenstein, CSW, Jenny Steingruebner, CTRS, Jerry Bruno, Janice Pelt, Trisha Lollo, and Andrea Horsch, RN. The book was also enhanced by the parent and patient commentary found throughout the text. We graciously thank Joan Jubela, Deborah Gordon, Annabel Wheeler, John and Catherine London, Abbe and Brian Walter, Robert Trama Sr., Michelle Bogosian, and Thomas Waters, Jr. for their comments and review of the manuscript. Finally, we would like to thank and commend Melissa Bruno for her invaluable contribution to this book. Her detailed drawings and graphics brought many of our explanations to life.

William L. Carroll, MD
Jessica B. Reisman, CSW
June, 2004

Dedication

Special thanks are also extended to my parents, Leslie and Steven; my sister Andrea; Zach; my in-laws Monte and Margery; and my sister-in-law, Courtney. They were tireless supporters and advocates, cheering me on to completion. Finally, I want to thank my partner and biggest fan: my husband, Adam. His never-ending faith and concise editing skills helped to turn this book into the reality you read today.

This book is dedicated to the memory of a special pink angel.

JR

This book is dedicated to my wife Saba and my five wonderful children, Bryan, Brenden, Michelle, Thomas, and Will, for their steadfast support of my career.

WLC

PART ONE

The Basics

What is cancer?

What causes cancer?

What is a tumor?

More ...

Cancer is a disease that affects not only the patient, but his or her family and friends as well. It is a disease with physical, social, emotional, financial, and psychological consequences, and education is an effective tool in combating its effects. Basic research has led to a much better understanding of human cancer in recent years. This chapter will identify basic terminology and concepts that are fundamental to a diagnosis of cancer.

1. What is cancer?

Cancer is a disease in which there is an abnormal, uncontrolled growth of cells or tissue. The human body is made up of billions of cells, each of which is programmed to perform a special function. Normal cells tend to grow and mature, and when their function is complete, they die. Therefore, the body is constantly replacing old cells with new cells in a tightly controlled manner. This natural process of cell growth, maturation, and death is impaired in cancer so that cancer cells grow no matter what signals they receive. Cancer cells can invade the surrounding tissues or organs, and then spread to distant sites in the body.

2. What causes cancer?

Growth is an important part of the body's metabolism. When a normal cell divides, it reproduces itself exactly. In the middle of the cell (the cell nucleus) are the **chromosomes**—delicate, double-helix–shaped filaments that hold all of the **genes** in place. Genes act to control the cell's behavior. Every gene is located in its own special place (**locus**) on the chromosome.

Chromosomes

strands that hold all of the genes in place.

Gene

Functional unit of heredity on a specific place (locus) on the chromosome; capable of reproducing itself exactly at each cell division; directs the formation of an enzyme or other protein.

Locus

a particular spot on a chromosome occupied by a specific gene.

Cancer cells do not respond to the same signals that control normal growth. They continue to grow despite indications (i.e., biochemical signals) to stop growing. Cancer occurs when a single cell in the body develops a mistake, called a **mutation**, in a gene (part of the DNA) that controls growth. The mutation leads to a growth signal that cannot be stopped. An individual cell probably needs to have five or six mutations in order for it to become truly cancerous. This is why cancer is relatively rare in children, whereas it is more common in older people: it takes time for cells to accumulate this damage to the DNA.

Scientists are constantly searching for clues that would indicate that some cases of childhood cancer might be linked to exposure to certain materials. Toxic material in the environment (called **carcinogens**), such as sun exposure or cigarette smoke, can cause an increase in mutations to DNA. However, these do not appear to play a significant role in childhood cancer.

There are very rare cases in which a cancer mutation may be passed from a parent to his or her child (**inherited mutation**). For example, certain forms of the common childhood eye cancer, called retinoblastoma, might be caused by an inherited mutation. However, the overwhelming majority of cases of childhood cancer are not inherited or due to environmental factors. In children these mistakes or mutations probably happen by accident, when normal cells double their DNA and their genes during cell division.

Cancer cells do not respond to the same signals that control normal growth.

The Basics

Mutation
a change in form of a gene.

Carcinogen
a toxic material in the environment known to cause cancer.

Inherited mutation
a mutation passed from a parent to his or her child.

Tumor

An abnormal
swelling, growth, or
mass (neoplasm) of
tissue in the body;
may be liquid (blood)
or solid (dense
mass), and benign
(does not form
metastases, and does
not invade or destroy
adjacent tissue) or
malignant (invades
surrounding tissues,
capable of producing
metastases, and may
recur after attempted
removal; likely to
cause death if left
untreated).

Benign

non-cancerous;
incapable of spread-
ing to other parts of
the body.

Malignant

cancerous; capable of
infiltrating locations
distant from the
place it originated.

Metastasize

the spread of cancer
cells from the original
site to colonize a
distant site.

3. What is a tumor?

A **tumor** refers to any abnormal growth or mass of tissue in the body. A parent or child might notice the tumor as it grows in size, or it may come to medical attention because of symptoms related to the tumor and/or its progression. For example, a bone tumor, which may not be visible to the eye, might cause destruction of normal bone and result in a fracture or pain.

The detection and/or presence of a tumor does not necessarily mean that it is cancerous (i.e., malignant; see Question 4). There are two types of tumors: liquid and solid. Leukemia, the most common cancer in children, is a cancer of the blood and therefore can be thought of as a "liquid tumor." Cancer can also appear as a solid mass, that is, a "solid tumor" such as bone cancer or brain cancer

4. What do the terms benign and malignant mean?

Tumors can be classified as **benign** or **malignant**. Benign refers to the fact that the tumor will not invade surrounding organs, nor will it spread (**metastasize**) to other parts of the body. Benign tumors can be removed surgically, and they will usually never recur. If it does return, it will most likely recur locally in the area where it was first noted, not in another part of the body. Under the microscope these tumors appear "bland," without many actively dividing cells. Most benign tumors are not life-threatening. However, if they occur in a critical area like the brain, they may be quite serious. They can also "push" the surrounding normal tissue aside, thereby resulting in damage.

The terms "malignant" and "cancerous" mean the same thing. Malignant tumors can invade surrounding normal structures and spread throughout the body. These tumors require aggressive treatment to prevent them from causing great harm. Figure 1 on page 6 shows how tumor cells progress. A discussion of the different stages of cancer can be found in Question 16.

5. Are childhood cancers similar to adult cancers?

Cancers that occur in children are distinctly different from those that occur in adults. The most important difference is that treatment options are generally more effective in children than in adults.

Cancers in children usually occur in the "brick and mortar" of the body, that is, the supporting structures such as bone marrow, muscle, bone (skeleton), and lymph nodes. Thus, leukemias (which first appear in bone marrow and blood), lymphomas (which are in the lymph nodes), sarcomas (found in bone and muscle), and Wilm's tumor (in kidneys) are common childhood tumors. In addition, tumors of the nervous system (such as brain tumors and neuroblastoma) are also frequently found among the range of tumor types in children. All are discussed in the questions throughout this book.

Treatment options are generally moer effective in children than in adults.

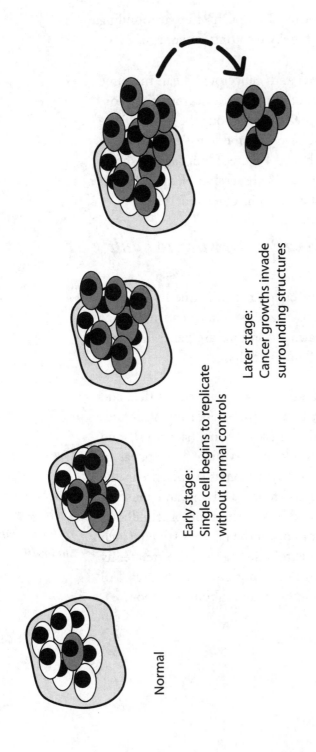

Normal

Early stage:
Single cell begins to replicate
without normal controls

Later stage:
Cancer growths invade
surrounding structures

Final stage:
Cancer cells travel to distant
sites within the body
(metastasis)

Figure 1.   Progression of cancer from normal to metastatic cancer.

In contrast, adult cancers often originate in the lining of organs, such as the gastrointestinal tract, lung, breast, and so forth, and are called carcinomas. Carcinomas are very rare in children. Figure 2 shows which childhood cancers are most common; the different types are described in the following special feature.

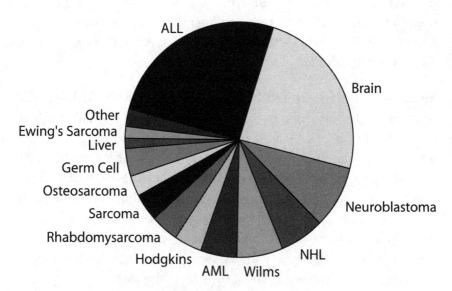

Figure 2. Common childhood cancers. Pie chart showing relative frequency of different cancers.

Common Cancers of Children

Acute Lymphoblastic Leukemia

Incidence: Acute lymphoblastic leukemia or ALL is the most common childhood cancer accounting for close to one third of all cancers in children. It is a cancer of the blood meaning that it starts in the bone marrow. Tumor cells, called **blasts**, circulate in the bloodstream. The peak incidence of ALL is between 2 to 5 years of age. Although exposure to irradiation has been associated with an increased risk of leukemia, there is no convincing evidence that routine x-rays play a role in childhood ALL. There is great interest in discovering possible environmental and viral causes of ALL, but there is no information currently to suggest that these exposures play a major role in most cases of ALL. Likewise, except for rare cases, ALL is not hereditary.

Symptoms, Diagnosis and Staging:[1] Children with ALL usually come to medical attention because of fatigue (due to anemia), bruising (a result of low platelets), bone pain (because of blast expansion in the bone marrow) and fever (due to infection because of low numbers of normal infection-fighting cells or due to the disease itself). Since blasts "crowd out" normal bone marrow cells, laboratory evaluation reveals low levels of normal blood cells: red cells, platelets, and normal white cells. In some cases leukemic blasts may be detected in the bloodstream. In addition, children with ALL may have enlarged lymph nodes or an enlargement of the liver and spleen.

There are two basic types of ALL, T-cell ALL and precursor B cell ALL. There are minor variations of the B type including B cell ALL that is really an advanced stage of Burkitt lymphoma (see Non-Hodgkin Lymphoma later in this section). Leukemias are not staged like solid tumors but risk factors have been identified that correlate

---

[1]For a discussion of cancer staging, see Question 16.

with the likelihood of cure. Patients who have blasts present in the spinal fluid (the natural fluid that surrounds the brain and spinal cord), and boys who have disease in the testes have a greater risk of relapse and therefore require extra treatment. In addition, children older than 10 and infants, as well as those with higher white blood cell counts at diagnosis (greater than 50,000 per microliter of blood), have a more aggressive type of leukemia and also need more intensified treatment. Genetic changes in the blasts themselves also dictate the degree of difficulty in curing the disease. For example, blasts that contain extra chromosomes (more than the standard 46 chromosomes, a condition called **hyperdiploidy**) are easier to cure compared to patients whose blasts contain fewer chromosomes. Translocations are abnormal fusions between different chromosomes, and they are often observed in blasts. Some translocations are "good," meaning that they are associated with a favorable cure rate. A common such translocation is called the TEL-AML 1 translocation. It is present in 25% of the precursor B cases. Unfavorable translocations include the "Philadelphia chromosome" (called Ph+) and "MLL" translocations. These latter patients may require additional therapy, including bone marrow transplantation in some cases.

Treatment: The treatment of leukemia involves the use of multiple drugs given in combination and in a particular sequence. These drugs are given by mouth, into the vein (IV), and into the spinal fluid (IT). Therapy is given in blocks designed to be more intense initially to prevent the disease from becoming resistant to treatment. The drugs given in induction, consolidation/central nervous system prophylaxis, interim maintenance, delayed intensification, and maintenance tend to vary; again, these are designed to maximize eradication of the leukemia and prevent any resistant tumor cells from developing.

For the more common B precursor ALL, girls are treated for a little over two years while boys are treated for an additional year. Therapy tends to be more intense early, but most of the treatment takes place in the doctor's office and by giving medications at home. Physicians will monitor how quickly the blasts disappear from the blood and/or bone marrow within the first few weeks after therapy is started to determine how sensitive the leukemia is to treatment. Sometimes treatment might be intensified if the number of leukemia cells disappears too slowly. T-cell ALL treatment usually consists of more intensified therapy, as is the case for infants. Cranial irradiation is not used for therapy in most cases of ALL but may be used if disease is present in the spinal fluid at diagnosis, for patients who have a very slow response to therapy, for children with T-cell ALL, and for patients who have a relapse. Bone marrow transplantation is reserved for patients with ALL and unfavorable features like Ph+ ALL or for those who suffer a relapse, especially if it occurs while still on treatment (called "early" relapse).

Acute and Chronic Myelogenous Leukemia

Incidence: Acute myelogenous leukemia or AML accounts for approximately 5% of all childhood cancers. It is a blood cancer like ALL but the blasts are "myeloid," meaning that they originated from a cell that was destined to develop into a neutrophil or monocyte as opposed to a lymphocyte. In adults, AML is the more common type of leukemia whereas ALL is more common in children. The cause of AML in most cases is unknown, although previous exposure to large doses of irradiation, benzenes, and chemotherapy has been associated with subsequent development of AML. Children with Down's syndrome have an increased risk of leukemia, both ALL and AML. Chronic myeloid leukemia (CML) is relatively rare in children and is usually like the "adult type" CML. Another rare type of leukemia called juvenile chronic myelomonocytic leukemia (JMML) can occur in younger children.

Symptoms, Diagnosis, and Staging: Children with AML usually see their doctor because of symptoms brought on by low blood counts. Like ALL, AML starts in the bone marrow, and the growth of the leukemia replaces the normal bone marrow. Therefore, the children experience fatigue and have a history of pallor (being pale due to anemia), easy bruising, nose bleeds, bleeding from the gums, and fever. Usually children with AML do not have extremely large lymph nodes or a large liver or spleen, which can be seen in ALL.

The diagnosis of AML is usually made by inspection of the blood and/or bone marrow. AML, being leukemia, is not staged like solid tumors. There are seven different subtypes (M1 through M7) of AML that can be distinguished by the way the cells look microscopically and the type of proteins expressed on the blast cell surface. Certain genetic changes can be seen in the leukemia; these "mutations" are unique to the leukemia and are not present in the normal cells/tissues of the body. The most common genetic changes involve two chromosomes joining together to form a translocation. The most common translocations are t(15;17) (meaning that chromosome 15 and chromosome 17 are now spliced together), t(8;21), and t(9;11). Sometimes AML cells may gain or lose a chromosome so that missing copies of chromosomes 7 and 5 may be detected or an extra copy of chromosome 8. The t(8;21) is commonly seen in the M2 subtype while the t(15;17) is seen in the M3 subtype of AML.

CML is a disease characterized by a smoldering "chronic phase" that lasts two to three years, followed by an "accelerated phase" that transitions into acute leukemia (called the "blast phase," either AML or ALL). Most patients are first diagnosed in the chronic phase with a very high white blood cell count and a very large spleen. Children with JMML usually have a skin rash, a large spleen, and low platelets on laboratory evaluation.

Treatment: Initial therapy for AML consists of one to two cycles of intensely applied chemotherapy to induce "remission." Because the dose and schedule of the chemotherapy is intense (to eradicate the more resistant AML cells) a prolonged recovery phase can be associated with severe infections and bleeding. The induction phase can last 4 to 6 weeks. Bone marrow transplantation has been shown to improve the cure rate for AML (from approximately 40–50% to 60–70%). However, only 25% of children will have a suitable donor. Induction is followed by either transplantation or further chemotherapy. The total treatment phase tends to be short (six to eight months) compared to the two to three years commonly used for ALL.

Treatment for acute promyelocytic leukemia (APL or the "M3" variant containing the t(15;17)) is unique in that the disease is responsive to therapy with all-trans-retinoic acid (ATRA), a form of vitamin A. Although ATRA is not curative by itself, when used with chemotherapy it is very effective. Because of the high cure rate, children with APL do not benefit from bone marrow transplantation unless the disease relapses. Arsenic is another compound that has been shown to be remarkably effective in treating APL.

The only curative therapy for CML in the past has been bone marrow transplantation. However, a new drug called imatinib has been designed that specifically disrupts the growth signal that results from the Philadelphia chromosome. The drug by itself is capable of inducing a remission when given in the chronic phase but resistance can occur. JMML responds to chemotherapy but BMT appears to be the best option for cure.

Non-Hodgkin Lymphoma

Incidence: Lymphomas are cancers of immune organs such as lymph nodes, the spleen, and the thymus (a very specialized immune organ next to the heart). They do not originate in the bone marrow like leukemias but can spread to the bone marrow. Therefore, lymphomas and leukemias are in the same family of cancers called hematopoie tumors. Collectively, lymphomas are the third most common cancer that occurs in children (after leukemia and brain tumors). Two thirds of lymphomas are of the non-Hodgkin lymphoma (NHL) type and one third are Hodgkin disease (see below). NHL can occur in children who suffer from a dysfunctional immune system, including patients on drugs used to prevent rejection after a solid organ or bone marrow transplant.

Symptoms, Diagnosis, and Staging: Children with lymphoma usually come to medical attention because of a persistently enlarged lymph node, often in the neck area. Other common symptoms include abdominal discomfort due to intestinal blockage from lymphoma or a chronic cough due to an enlarged mass in the thymus that impinges on airways in the chest. The diagnosis is made by a biopsy (see Question 14) of the mass in question.

There are three main types of childhood NHL: Burkitt (50% of NHL), lymphoblastic (40%), and large cell (20%). The Burkitt type usually occurs in the intestine or back of the mouth (pharynx) whereas lymphoblastic lymphomas characteristically are associated with enlargement of lymph nodes in the neck area and the thymus gland in the chest. Large-cell lymphomas can occur anywhere in the body and are further subdivided into large B-cell lymphoma and anaplastic large-cell lymphoma (T cell).

Lymphomas are staged according to the number of sites involved. Stages I and II refer to either a single site or two adjacent sites respectively. All large tumors and those NHLs that involve two sites distant from one another are classified as stage III. Stage IV disease either involves the bone marrow and/or the spinal fluid.

Treatment: Chemotherapy is used to treat lymphomas. The types of drugs and the duration depend on the type of NHL and the stage. Localized NHL (stages I and II) may require as little as three months of treatment. Advanced stage Burkitt and large B-cell lymphoma responds best to 6 to 8 months of aggressive "pulse" treatment whereas lymphoblastic lymphoma is treated a lot like ALL (see above). Radiation therapy is usually not needed, and bone marrow transplantation is reserved only for patients who relapse. Cure rates for localized NHL are above 90%, while those for advanced disease are approximately 75% to 80%.

Hodgkin Disease

Incidence: Hodgkin disease (HD) has a tendency to occur in adolescence/young adulthood and in patients over 50 years of age. Males are more prone to the disease than females. Studies suggest that HD may be linked to environmental factors and/or hereditary factors. HD in young children is more common in patients with lower socioeconomic status, whereas in adolescents it is more common in Caucasians. Family members of patients with HD also seem to be at greater risk of getting the disease, although in practical terms the chance that a brother or sister will also get HD is very remote. These observations have led doctors to conclude that HD may be linked to an infectious agent. The Epstein-Barr virus (the virus that causes mononucleosis) has been linked to HD, but its exact role in the disease is still uncertain.

Symptoms, Diagnosis, and Staging: Children with HD often have a history of painless swollen lymph nodes that are unresponsive to antibiotics. More than two thirds of HD cases occur in the neck area and often there is enlargement of the thymus (like NHL, see above).

Close to a third of children will have associated symptoms of fever, night sweats, and weight loss (so-called "B" symptoms). The diagnosis is made by lymph node biopsy. Although multiple different forms of HD can be distinguished by microscopic appearance they all respond to therapy identically except for the "lymphocyte predominant" form, which has the best prognosis. Staging for HD is a lot like NHL with stages I and II referring to a single or two closely associated areas of involvement respectively. Stage III refers to involvement of lymph nodes on both sides of the diaphragm, which separates the chest from the abdomen. Stage IV is used to classify patients who have widespread involvement outside the lymph nodes, including the bone marrow and liver.

Treatment: Classically, radiation therapy (RT) was used to treat patients with localized disease, and most patients can be cured with this approach. However, chemotherapy is needed for patients with more advanced disease. Chemotherapy is now used routinely in children, even for localized disease, since the dose of RT needed to cure HD is quite high, causing growth inhibition of soft tissues and bones. Thus most modern protocols rely on chemotherapy, often combined with lower dose RT. Treatment usually consists of 4 to 6 or more cycles of chemotherapy lasting 6 to 8 months. HD is one of the most curable of all human cancers with cure rates of 90 to 100% for localized disease (stages I and II) and 75 to 90% for advanced disease. Since the cure rate for HD is so high, there is a great emphasis on developing new protocols that are associated with fewer long-term side effects like infertility and second tumors.

Brain Tumors

Incidence: Brain tumors are the second most common cancer in children (after ALL), accounting for 20% of all new cases of cancer in children. Children with certain inherited conditions such as neurofibromatosis are at greater risk for developing a brain tumor.

Although no clear environmental risk factor is present, in most cases the incidence of brain tumors appears to be increasing. In part, this increase may be artificial due to better radiographic techniques capable of detecting tumors at an earlier stage. Previous radiation therapy to the head area, like that used to treat certain types of leukemia in the past, has been linked to subsequent development of brain tumors.

Symptoms, Diagnosis, and Staging: There are many different types of brain tumors, each of which can be slow growing (so-called "low grade" tumors) or more rapidly growing ("high-grade"). A complete description of all types of brain tumors is beyond the scope of this book. Symptoms are usually related to the site of origin. Many tumors lead to increased pressure in the brain, a condition called hydrocephalus, that occurs as a result of blockage to craniospinal fluid flow. Such patients have increasing headache (that may be especially severe in the early morning hours), vomiting, irritability, and double vision. Tumors that arise in the back of the brain may cause imbalance and difficulty walking. Young infants with brain tumors may show loss of certain milestones and irritability. Finally, symptoms of tumors that start in the upper parts of the brain include headaches, seizures, and weakness.

The diagnosis of a brain tumor is usually made by magnetic resonance imaging (MRI) or computed tomography (CT) imaging. Although the CT scan can detect most tumors, MRI is preferable because it is a more sensitive technique. Staging for brain tumors takes into consideration the size of the mass and whether it has spread to other parts of the brain and spinal cord. After a tumor is visualized in the brain it is also important to examine the spinal canal with MRI to determine whether additional spread has occurred. Only rarely do brain tumors spread outside the nervous system. A biopsy and possible surgical resection establish the exact diagnosis. In some cases a biopsy may be hazardous because of possible collateral damage to normal nerve tissue. Brainstem tumors (e.g. the base of the brain) like gliomas may be diagnosed by MRI, thereby avoiding a risky surgery.

Treatment: Most brain tumors are localized at diagnosis, and complete surgical removal would be the desired goal. However, two important features may limit their complete resection. First, it is often difficult to define a clear margin of separation between malignant and normal tissues. Many brain tumors infiltrate tissue rather than pushing surrounding normal nervous tissue aside. Therefore, it is difficult for the surgeon to be certain that the tumor is completely removed. Second, given the importance of brain structures, it is often impossible to remove the tumor completely without causing significant and permanent brain damage.

Radiation therapy has been used for many years to treat brain tumors and remains one of the most effective forms of treatment. However, because of significant neuropsychological side effects oncologists may be reluctant to use this form of treatment, especially in infants. Newer techniques such as three-dimensional conformal radiotherapy and intensity modulated radiotherapy are now available that allow doctors to deliver radiation more precisely, thereby sparing surrounding normal brain. Chemotherapy is being used with increasing frequency. This has led to improved cure rates for many tumors such as medulloblastoma, "PNET" tumors, germ cell tumors, and more recently for some gliomas. In some cases, chemotherapy improves tumor kill so that the dose of radiation can be reduced (with reduced side effects), delayed until the child reaches an age where side effects are less severe, or eliminated completely.

Neuroblastoma

Incidence: Neuroblastoma is the second most common solid tumor in children, accounting for up to 10% of cancers. The cause of neuroblastoma is unknown, and there is little evidence that environmental factors play a role. Heredity has been implicated in some cases since the disease can run in families, although this is rare. The tumor originates in parts of the nervous system called the peripheral nervous system, referring to areas outside of the brain and spinal cord. Neuroblastoma usually starts in the adrenal gland, which lies in the abdomen, but neuroblastoma can also occur in the chest, pelvis, and other sites.

Symptoms, Diagnosis, and Staging: Tumors of the abdomen can be associated with pain, and often parents might feel a hard mass in the area. Neuroblastomas that occur next to the spine may impinge on nerves, so weakness and numbness of the legs might occur along with difficulty urinating or loss of bowel control. Since many neuroblastomas have spread to other parts of the body (liver, bones, bone marrow, lymph nodes, and skin) patients may have a history of irritability (due to bone pain) and weight loss (due to general side effects of the tumor). These tumors have a tendency to metastasize to the bones that surround the eyes, so children may develop bruising in this area. A rare condition called opsomyoclonus, which consists of rapid "darting" eye movements, may signal neuroblastoma.

CT/MRI scans usually reveal a typical appearance of neuroblastoma. Additional tests like bone scans, bone marrow aspirates and bone marrow biopsies are done to determine whether the tumor has spread. A positive result for a special test called an MIBG scan indicates neuroblastoma in most cases. Another clue to the diagnosis can come from analysis of substances called "catecholamines" that are substances made by neuroblastoma tumor cells. Catecholamines (called "HVA" and "VMA") are measured in the urine, and doctors will measure them periodically during treatment since levels should return to normal if the tumor is completely cured. The final diagnosis of neuroblastoma is made by microscopic examination of a biopsy sample. Neuroblastomas have three different appearances under the microscope. The most common type is *neuroblastoma,* which is the most malignant form, and here there are two subtypes: "favorable" (e.g. easier to treat) and "unfavorable." *Ganglioneuroblastoma* refers to a tumor that is a mixture of malignant and benign tumor cells whereas *ganglioneuroma* is a benign form of neuroblastoma.

Neuroblastomas are staged like other solid tumors: Stage 1 includes tumors that are completely removed at diagnosis; stage 2 characterizes tumors that are removed surgically but small amounts of tumor (detected by microscopic examination of the surgical sample) are left behind; stage 3 means tumors that are localized but are so big and/or encase normal organs such that they cannot be surgically resected; and stage 4 refers to patients whose tumors have spread distantly to other parts of the body. A very special stage called stage 4S refers to young infants (less than one year old) who have a very small "primary" tumor along with disease that may be in the bone marrow, liver, or skin, but not in the bone itself. Curiously, these tumors may disappear completely on their own without any therapy.

Treatment: Many characteristics help doctors decide the best treatment for neuroblastoma. Certainly the stage of the tumor helps since stages 1 and 2 tumors may require surgery alone while stages 3 and 4 tumors need chemotherapy. Age is also important since young children (less than 12 to 18 months of age) have a higher cure rate than older children. Laboratory analysis of the tumor itself also provides clues as to how curable a particular neuroblastoma is. For example, extra copies of chromosomes signals a more curable tumor in infants while extra copies of a particular gene called "N-myc" means that the neuroblastoma is less curable. However, all of these factors are not 100% predictive and monitoring how the tumor responds to treatment (e.g. how it shrinks after therapy is started) is one of the best ways to determine how curable a particular tumor is.

Most cases of neuroblastoma require chemotherapy, and treatment plans contain a number of medications. After chemotherapy is used to shrink tumors, surgical resection may be possible to remove remaining tumor not killed by chemotherapy. The surgery is usually followed by more chemotherapy, which attacks tumor cells present in other parts of the body. In addition, neuroblastomas are sensitive to radiation treatment, which is often used in combination with surgery and chemotherapy. Stage 4 tumors in older children are more difficult to treat since the tumor may be only partially sensitive to the above measures. Using high-dose chemotherapy with autologous bone marrow transplantation (e.g. using the patient's own bone marrow) has been shown to be effective for this form of neuroblastoma. Another complementary form of therapy relies on using a form of vitamin A called *cis* retinoic acid. This medication directs remaining cancer cells to change from malignant cells to a benign form that is harmless.

Like other forms of childhood cancer, many new treatments are currently being evaluated for neuroblastoma. A particularly promising approach is the use of monoclonal antibodies that bind to tumor cells and kill them through the immune system.

Osteosarcoma
Incidence: Osteosarcoma is the most common bone tumor in children and frequently occurs in adolescents. The cause is unknown in most cases. Prior radiation therapy (to treat a previ-

ous tumor) and a rare hereditary syndrome called Li-Fraumeni syndrome are associated with an increased risk of developing osteosarcoma.

Symptoms, Diagnosis, and Staging: Children with osteosarcoma often have a history of pain and swelling at the tumor site. While the onset of symptoms may be related to a fall or sports injury, trauma is not known to be a cause of osteosarcoma. Most tumors occur at the ends of bones, most often around the knee (e.g. in the femur or tibia). X-rays usually show bone destruction. An MRI will reveal the full extent of the tumor, including any growth of the tumor into surrounding tissues. Most tumors are localized at diagnosis but approximately 25% of patients may have disease that has spread to other areas in the body. The lungs are the most common site of metastasis (90%) followed by involvement of other bones. A CT scan of the chest and bone scan can determine whether the disease has spread to other areas. Staging in osteosarcoma is based on whether the tumor is localized or has metastasized.

Treatment: The only way to cure osteosarcoma is to totally remove the tumor surgically. It does not respond well to radiation treatments. However even with complete removal many tumors will recur, especially in the lungs. Initial surgical removal may be difficult if the tumor is large. Currently chemotherapy is used first to shrink the tumor and to kill any tumor cells that may have spread to other areas at diagnosis. After approximately 12 weeks of chemotherapy, the surgeon removes the tumor and in most cases the bone can be reconstructed. Amputation is done much less frequently given improvements in surgical techniques. After the tumor is removed, the amount of living vs. dead ("necrotic") tumor cells is evaluated by looking at the sample under the microscope. If the sample shows that very little tumor is remaining (e.g. most of the tumor is dead or necrotic), the outlook for cure is much better.

After the tumor is removed, another six months or so of treatment is given to be sure that the child is completely cured. If the tumor is localized when first detected, the chance for complete cure is approximately 70%, whereas tumors that show spread to the lungs, or other bones are harder to treat (25 to 30% cure rate).

Ewing Sarcoma

Incidence: Ewing sarcoma is the second most common bone children and, like osteosarcoma, often occurs in adolescents. In addition to its location in bones, it can also occur in the "soft tissues" of the body near muscles. Another version of Ewing sarcoma is called "PNET." The exact cause of Ewing tumor is not known. It is not hereditary, although is uncommon in black and Asian children. A genetic mutation called a translocation involving chromosome 22 is observed in tumor cells (not in normal cells in the body) but this mutation has not been linked to exposure to environmental toxins.

Symptoms, Staging, and Diagnosis: Pain and swelling are the most common symptoms that bring the child to the doctor. Ewing tumors can occur in any bone, but in contrast to osteosarcomas usually develop in the middle of long bones rather than the ends. If the tumor is particularly large or if the tumor has spread to other areas the parents may note fever and weight loss. The diagnosis can be suspected if x-rays show destruction of normal bone and/or a mass. This finding is confirmed by a CT scan or MRI scan. Ewing tumors can spread to the lungs, other bones, or bone marrow so a CT scan of the chest as well as bone scan and bone marrow biopsies/aspirates are all part of the initial battery of tests that needs to be done (see Questions 17 and 18).

The actual diagnosis is made by a biopsy, in which microscopic examination by a pathologist shows the typical microscopic appearance of Ewing tumor. There is no formal staging system in Ewing sarcoma other than whether the disease is localized or metastatic. Patients with smaller tumors (less than 5 cm) do better than those who have larger tumors, but the majority of children with localized disease are cured (approximately 65 to 70% cure rate). Children with metastatic disease do not do as well, although those patients with pulmonary metastasis fare better than children who have tumor cells in other areas like the bone marrow.

Treatment: The treatment of Ewing sarcoma is directed against the primary tumor using surgery and/or radiation therapy as well as chemotherapy to kill cancer cells that may have spread. Usually chemotherapy is administered first because this approach has the added advantage of shrinking the tumor so that it can be removed completely with minimal damage to surrounding normal structures. The resected tumor can be examined microscopically to determine how effective the initial treatment was against the cancer cells. Patients whose tumors show the greatest amount of tumor kill (necrosis) have the best outcome. Following surgery, further chemotherapy is given so that the patient has the greatest chance of cure. The total duration of therapy is usually a little less than a full year. Children with localized Ewing tumors have a 70% cure, while patients with metastasis do poorly. Newer approaches are evaluating whether high-dose chemotherapy followed by autologous bone marrow transplantation improves outcome for patients with highly refractory or metastatic Ewing tumor.

Wilms Tumor

Incidence: Wilms tumor is the most common kidney tumor of children. It usually occurs in one kidney, although some patients have tumors in both kidneys. Wilms tumor commonly occurs in children between 3 and 5 years of age, and at a younger age with bilateral tumors. Like other childhood cancers, the cause of most cases of Wilms tumor is unknown. It is more likely to develop in patients who have rare developmental syndromes (Denys-Drash, Beckwith-Wiedeman, and WAGR syndromes) but the overwhelming number of children with Wilms tumor do not have these syndromes.

Symptoms, Diagnosis, and Staging: Most children are diagnosed because parents notice abdominal swelling or actually feel a mass in the abdomen. Many children have no symptoms, but pain, blood in the urine, and fever may be present. Radiographic evaluation by ultrasound or CT usually shows the typical appearance of a mass originating in the kidney (as opposed to a neuroblastoma, which originates in the adrenal gland located just above the kidneys). Wilms tumors can spread to the lungs, so a CT of the chest is also done as part of the evaluation. The diagnosis is established by microscopic evaluation of a surgical sample of the tumor (see below). Most patients have a typical Wilms tumor when the pathologist examines the microscopic appearance, but about 5% of patients have "anaplastic" subtypes that require more treatment. In addition, there are two other kidney tumors, clear cell sarcoma and rhabdoid tumor, which are associated with a worse outcome compared to Wilms tumor. Staging is as follows: Stage I—completely removed by surgery; stage II—the tumor extends beyond the kidney but is removed by surgery completely; stage III—the tumor is localized to the kidney area but cannot be removed completely; stage IV—metastatic tumor in lungs, distant lymph nodes or liver; and stage V—tumor in both kidneys.

Treatment: Most Wilms tumors can be removed surgically at diagnosis. Patients are treated with a short course of chemotherapy to be certain that any tumor cells that are left behind or present elsewhere in the body are killed. Treatment is short for patients with stage I and II tumors, consisting of two drugs administered for just over 4 months. A low dose of radiation to the tumor plus an additional drug is used to treat stage III tumors while additional drugs and low-dose radiation to the lungs may be given for patients with stage IV Wilms tumors. Outcome for Wilms tumor is outstanding, with greater than a 90% cure rate for stages I to III, and approximately 80% for stage IV.

Rhabdomyosarcoma

Incidence: Rhabdomyosarcomas are tumors of muscle tissue and account for 5% of all childhood cancers. The cause of rhabdomyosarcoma is not known.

Symptoms, Diagnosis, and Staging: Rhabdomyosarcomas can develop anywhere skeletal muscle tissue is present and therefore symptoms are related to the location of the primary tumor. Older children tend to have tumors that start in the arms or legs, and symptoms consist of an enlarging mass or lump. Rhabdomyosarcomas of the head and neck may start as a lump or may cause headaches, sinus congestion, or local nerve dysfunction. Tumors of the pelvis may cause pain and bladder dysfunction.

A CT or MRI shows a "soft tissue" mass (as opposed to a bone tumor). Since the tumor can travel to the lungs, bones, and bone marrow, a CT scan of the chest, bone scan, and bone marrow biopsy/aspirate are done when rhabdomyosarcoma is suspected. The diagnosis is established when microscopic examination of a surgical sample is done. There are two main types of rhabdomyosarcoma: "alveolar" and "embryonal." Embryonal tumors are easier to treat. Alveolar rhabdomyosarcomas are characterized by translocations involving genes called "PAX" and "FKHR."

Rhabdomyosarcomas are classified by a complex staging system that depends on size, location, and whether the tumor can be removed by surgery. For example, the tumors are "grouped" the following way: Group I—localized tumor, completely removed surgically; group II—localized tumor completely removed surgically but when the sample is examined under the microscope the pathologist determines that a small amount of tumor may still be present in the body; group III—surgery is not possible because the tumor is too large or involves surrounding normal tissue in such a way that surgery would cause significant damage; and group IV—rhabdomyosaromas that show evidence of distant metastasis. "Stage" for rhabdomyosarcoma refers to location, the size of the tumor, and whether lymph nodes are involved. Thus, each tumor is defined by a group and a stage.

Treatment: Rhabdomyosarcomas are treated with a combination of surgery, radiation, and chemotherapy. For tumors that are completely removed, chemotherapy is used to kill remaining tumor cells that may be "hiding" in other parts of the body (e.g. lungs). Chemotherapy may also be used to shrink large tumors so that they can be fully removed at a "second look" surgery 10 to 12 weeks later. If the primary tumor cannot be removed, then radiation therapy is used to treat the primary tumor in addition to chemotherapy. The cure rate for rhabdomyosarcoma ranges from over 80% to less than 30% depending on whether the tumor is alveolar vs. embryonal type, and its stage and group. Embryonal tumors that are localized (especially if they are in certain locations, such as next to the eye, head, and neck) are very curable whereas alveolar tumors that have spread to other parts of the body (e.g. metastatic disease) are the most difficult to treat.

Liver tumors
Incidence: There are two basic types of liver tumors: a cancer called *hepatoblastoma* that usually occurs in infants, and a cancer

called *hepatocellular carcinoma* that is more common in older children and adults. Hepatocellular carcinomas can arise in diseased livers due to hepatitis. The cause of most hepatoblastomas is unknown, although rarely they can occur in children with certain genetic syndromes.

Symptoms: Most patients have a painless mass that is felt by parents or they notice an enlarging abdomen. Sometimes liver tumors may cause pain, fever, or jaundice. A CT or MRI scan can show one or more tumors in the liver. Most liver tumors produce a factor called alpha fetoprotein and high levels of AFP indicate the presence of a liver tumor or a germ cell tumor (see below). Since liver tumors may also travel to the lungs a CT scan of this area is warranted also. Staging is similar to other solid tumors.

Treatment: The only way to cure liver tumors is to surgically remove them. If this is not possible at diagnosis, chemotherapy can be used to shrink the tumor so it can be removed completely. Hepatoblastomas are sensitive to chemotherapy, but chemotherapy alone cannot cure hepatoblastoma. The speed at which high AFP levels return to normal can be used to follow the effectiveness of treatment. If the tumor cannot be removed even after receiving chemotherapy, liver transplantation can be considered. Tumors that show evidence of disease that has traveled to the lungs are very difficult to treat. Hepatocellular carcinoma does not respond to chemotherapy well, so surgical removal is quite important in this disease also.

Germ Cell Tumors

Incidence: Germ cell tumors account for 3% of all childhood cancers. They originate in cells that were used in fetal life to give rise to the ovaries and testes. Germ cell tumors of adults usually occur in the ovary or the testis, but in children they are more likely to occur in cells that were in the process of migrating during fetal life to the ovaries or testes. They can occur anywhere, in the brain, chest, abdomen, ovary, testes, or near the tail-bone. Two peaks of germ cell tumors are seen; in infancy and then again in adolescence. The cause of germ cell tumors is unknown, but male patients with an extra X chromosome are at greater risk.

Symptoms, Diagnosis, and Staging: Symptoms of germ cell tumors are related to location. For example germ cell tumors of the brain may be associated with headache, vomiting, imbalance, and double vision, while those that occur in the chest usually cause cough and difficulty breathing. Tumors of the ovary can result in pain and nausea because the cancer can lead to twisting of the blood supply. Newborns with germ cell tumors of the lower back will have an identifiable mass in the area, and testicular tumors also present with a lump.

Most germ cell tumors (like liver tumors) also produce alpha feto-protein and some produce another hormone, β-HCG, so that levels of these two substances can be detected in the blood. Radiographic tests such as CT or MRI will typically show a mass. Location in the brain or chest can be confused with other tumor types, while a few other tumors develop in the ovaries or testes. Germ cell tumors can be benign (called teratomas) or malignant, and the final diagnosis is established by a pathologist after examination of the tumor under the microscope.

Treatment: Benign germ cell tumors require surgery alone, while the malignant varieties require chemotherapy and on occasion radiation. Most malignant germ cell tumors are extremely sensitive to treatment, so even patients with advanced disease have a high likelihood of cure.

Histiocytosis

Incidence: Histiocytosis actually refers to two main disorders: *Langerhan's cell histiocytosis* or LCH, and *hemophagocytic lymphohistiocytosis* or HLH. Both tumors develop within types of white blood cells called mononuclear cells, and therefore these diseases are related to leukemia. Both LCH and HLH tend to occur in young children, often under one year of age. Although LCH has been known to occur within families, and some studies have linked the disease to some environmental exposures, most cases have no clear cause. HLH can occur in the setting of immune dysfunction and infection, especially with Epstein-Barr, the mononucleosis virus. There are also cases that are due to an inherited defect.

Symptoms, Diagnosis, and Staging: LCH can involve different sites within the body and therefore symptoms can be quite diverse. Sometimes it involves a single bone. Growth of the abnormal cells causes bone destruction, so pain and swelling may occur. It can also involve tissue around the eyes and destroy part of the pituitary gland, affecting the body's ability to regulate water retention by the kidneys. Children may complain of excessive thirst, or parents may note that the child is urinating excessively. A history of chronic draining ear infections, a persistent scalp rash, or bleeding from the gums may be present, all related to growth of the abnormal cells. Finally, a particularly severe form of LCH is seen in infants involving multiple organs, including the liver, spleen, lungs, skin, and bone marrow. These children appear very ill with a long history of poor feeding, irritability, a rash, and fever.

Children with HLH are usually quite sick when they come to medical attention. Widespread involvement of multiple organs is common, and the children have fever, weakness, and irritability. Examination shows enlargement of the liver, spleen, and lymph nodes. Since the bone marrow is often involved, blood counts are low, so anemia and easy bruising can be seen. Laboratory tests show liver dysfunction (jaundice) and high levels of triglycerides along with low levels of blood clotting factors.

Treatment: The treatment for LCH depends on how many areas are affected. Sometimes a simple surgical procedure to "curette" or scoop out the diseased portion of the bone may eradicate the LCH. Other chemotherapy drugs work also. The goal is to give drugs with the fewest side effects. Treatment is relatively easy compared to other forms of cancer, but severe forms do require more aggressive treatment. On the other hand, children with HLH are very sick and require prompt medical therapy. A combination of chemotherapy drugs and medicines that regulate the immune system (e.g. the same drugs that are used to prevent transplant organ rejection) are used to put HLH into remission. Since HLH may also involve the brain, drugs may also be given into the spinal fluid, again like the treatment that is used for other forms of leukemia. Children with the inherited form of HLH require bone marrow transplantation.

Retinoblastoma

Incidence: Retinoblastoma is the most common eye tumor in children. Two thirds of cases involve only one eye, but bilateral involvement occurs due to an inherited genetic defect in a gene called "Rb" (for retinoblastoma). Retinoblastoma is the only childhood tumor where heredity plays a big role. Children with involvement of both eyes tend to be younger when first diagnosed, and some cases are picked up because there is a family history of retinoblastoma.

Symptoms, Diagnosis, and Staging: The most common symptom is when parents or the primary pediatrician notice an abnormal light reflex in the eye. The light reflex appears white instead of the normal red reflex that occurs when a light is flashed in front of the eyes. The eye may also wander or not move in sync with the other eye. The diagnosis is established by an examination by an ophthalmologist with the child under anesthesia. A CT scan will document the size of the tumor and whether it actually involves the major nerve that supplies the eye. Retinoblastoma tumors are usually quite localized and rarely travel outside of the globe of the eye.

Treatment: Since almost all retinoblastomas are localized, the usual approach has been to remove the eye and replace it with a cosmetic artificial eye. This is still done if no useful vision is present in the affected eye. Historically, in cases of bilateral retinoblastoma the most severely affected eye was removed and radiation was used to treat the less severely affected eye. However, a major emphasis is now placed on using newer approaches to preserve vision in both eyes if at all possible. Therefore radiation, laser therapy, and cryotherapy (cold treatment) can be used to treat small tumors. However, radiation therapy can lead to second tumors in the radiation field and deformities to the growing bone, limiting its application. Chemotherapy is being used with greater frequency in an effort to shrink tumors, thereby preserving useful vision and preventing the need for surgical removal and/or irradiation of the eye. The cure rate for retinoblastoma is greater than 95%.

6. Is this our fault? What could we have done to prevent this from happening to our child?

At this time, there is no known cause of cancer in children. Nevertheless, guilt is a common parental emotion associated with a child's initial diagnosis. Parents or caregivers often feel that they should have been able to "protect" their child from the illness. Yet, at this time, there is nothing known that can be done to prevent pediatric cancers from occurring. Pediatric cancers have not been shown to be a result of what you fed your child, whom your child played with, or where you live. Although research continues to explore the origin of pediatric cancers, the question of "why" still remains. There is one thing that is clear—cancer is not a parent's fault.

Guilt is a common parental emotion associated with a child's initial diagnosis

"Don't waste your time on why; instead, focus on what you can do from here."

—Mother of a young child diagnosed with a brain tumor

7. Do our other children have a chance of getting cancer?

Cancer is not contagious. The illness cannot be "caught" by any means. However, there are some forms of cancer that may prove to have a hereditary component and have been documented in multiple family members. For example, the childhood eye tumor, retinoblastoma, may have a hereditary component. Genetic tests can determine if this is the case. Other cancer-prone diagnoses are extremely rare genetic syndromes.

PART TWO

Diagnosis

Our child is suspected of having cancer. What do we do next, and what can we anticipate?

Would it have made a difference if we had brought our child to the doctor sooner?

More ...

When cancer is suspected, there are three important questions that need to be addressed: 1) Is cancer present? 2) If cancer is the diagnosis, what is the type of cancer? and 3) What is the stage of the cancer? These questions are answered through a series of physical examinations by specialists, laboratory tests, imaging techniques, (e.g., x-rays and other tests), and often a surgical procedure called a biopsy.

8. Our child is suspected of having cancer. What do we do next, and what can we anticipate?

Seek a physician and facility that specialize in the care of children with cancer.

You should seek a physician and facility that specialize in the care of children with cancer. In addition to an experienced pediatric oncologist who is board certified (you can check by accessing the American Board of Pediatrics Web site at *www.abp.org*), you should look for a medical team that has experience dealing with all dimensions of therapy, including medical treatment (doctors, nurse practitioners, chemo-pharmacists, and nurses) as well as psychosocial issues (dedicated social workers, psychologists, child-life specialists, music therapists, etc.).

Arm yourself with knowledge.

Arm yourself with knowledge. Understanding basic terminology about the diagnosis will help you to feel more secure during this critical time. The Internet and educational resources, such as this book, can be a starting place for research, but all information should be reviewed with your chosen medical team. Medical advances are taking place rapidly and information in print or on the Web may be outdated. Education will be reinforced once your child begins treatment. You should expect to meet with the medical team frequently, and one or more extended sessions should be scheduled to review all results and treatment approaches. Feel confidence in your chosen medical team and seek a second opinion if you feel it is necessary.

"Keep a journal close at hand. When a question or thought comes up, write it down. Read through your questions to determine if they have a theme. Then decide who can be most helpful in answering your questions."

—Mother of a child diagnosed with a brain tumor

"Always ask for and read the written reports prepared by the doctors who are checking out your child. We have gone back (since diagnosis) and looked at the original paperwork and test results and found some clues to his diagnosis. The word 'leukemia' does come up (in some reports) a few times, but it wasn't imparted to us."

—Mother of a child diagnosed with leukemia

9. Would it have made a difference if we had brought our child to the doctor sooner?

It is unlikely that recognizing a cancer diagnosis a few weeks to months earlier would change the cure rate for most cancers. However, if some types of cancer are caught in their early stages, it may make a cure more likely. But, in general, coming to the doctor earlier would not have had a tremendous impact on the likelihood of cure. According to statistics, most general pediatricians make approximately one pediatric cancer diagnosis every 10 years. It often can be difficult for parents as well as some pediatricians to discern the early signs of an impending cancer diagnosis. Most of the initial presenting symptoms, especially with leukemia, appear to be consistent with fatigue, the flu, or the common cold. It is important to remember that pediatric cancer is a rare diagnosis. Also, current information indicates that most cancers develop a particular pattern of spread early, so that the stage of a particular cancer is determined early in the evolution of the disease. In other words, even if the clock could be turned back in time, it is unlikely that recognizing it a few weeks to months earlier would change the cure rate for most cancers.

"Our initial pediatrician was frustrated by our insistence that something was wrong. He blamed us and told us the symptoms our son was reporting were in his mind. Don't let them do that to you. Be persistent. You know when something isn't right with your child. If your child doesn't want to go outside and complains of pain, you know something is wrong, regardless of what a doctor may say."

—Mother of a child diagnosed with leukemia

---

10. What is leukemia?

Leukemia is the most common form of cancer found in children. It begins in the bone marrow. Bone marrow is the hollow internal scaffolding of bones where blood cells develop. When a child is diagnosed with leukemia, the normal bone marrow is usually replaced with leukemia cells that are called **blasts**. Since normal bone marrow is no longer functioning properly, the normal blood cells decline in number. Therefore, the child usually has a history of fatigue due to anemia and possibly bruising because of a low platelet count (see Question 13). Leukemia is often called a "liquid tumor." Instead of being a solid mass, individual tumor cells (all of which are identical to one another) travel throughout the body in the bloodstream.

Leukemia

a cancer of the bone marrow that is the most common cancer in children.

Blasts

immature blood cells.

There are many subtypes of leukemia, but the two main categories are acute lymphoblastic leukemia (ALL) and acute myelogenous leukemia (AML). ALL accounts for approximately 25% of all childhood cancers, making it the most common form. Among ALL cases there are subtypes based on whether it is a "T-cell" or a "precursor B-cell" ALL. Although the general approach may be similar, different types of ALL require different treatments.

AML is less common and occurs in approximately 5% of childhood cancer cases. Its treatment is quite different from that used in treating ALL. There are seven different types of AML, and even among these cases treatment could be different. For example, the M3 subtype of AML is called acute promyelocytic leukemia (APML) and is treated with vitamin A (trans-retinoic acid or ATRA) in addition to chemotherapy. Moreover, a bone marrow transplant, which is usually preferable in combination with conventional chemotherapy for AML, is not indicated in APML.

11. What is a lymphoma?

Lymphomas are cancers that start in lymph nodes. Lymph nodes are small pea-sized nodules that are present throughout the body and are normally composed of white blood cells. Lymph nodes act as filters to rid the body of germs, and they often enlarge during infections. For example, it is quite common to be able to feel lymph nodes at the angle of the jaw at the top of the neck ("cervical lymph nodes"), since throat infections are quite common, especially in children. However, when lymphomas develop, the lymph nodes become much larger because the normal lymph cells are completely

Lymphoma
cancer that starts in lymph nodes.

replaced by tumor cells, and frequently a number of adjacent lymph nodes become "matted" or adherent to one another. Lymphomas may also involve other sites, particularly the bone marrow, thymus (an immune system organ located in the chest), liver, and spleen.

There are two major types of lymphoma: Hodgkin disease and non-Hodgkin lymphoma (NHL). Lymphomas are closely related to leukemias, and in some cases the treatments are quite similar.

12. What is the difference between Hodgkin and non-Hodgkin lymphoma?

Hodgkin disease and non-Hodgkin lymphoma are the two major types of lymphoma, but they are quite different when it comes to treatment. Hodgkin disease is a lymphoma that spreads locally from one lymph node to an adjacent lymph node, whereas non-Hodgkin lymphoma (NHL) occurs in similar structures initially, but then quickly spreads through the blood. There are different subtypes of Hodgkin disease and non-Hodgkin lymphomas based on their microscopic appearance. The types and duration of treatment depend on the subtype and the stage of the disease (see the Special Feature in Part One).

13. What is a CBC and how is it read?

The most routine laboratory test that will be done during treatment is called a **complete blood count** or CBC. This test measures the cells present in the blood. There are three basic types of cells that circulate in the blood: **red blood cells**, **white blood cells**, and **platelets**. Each type is suited to a particular task, and all are affected by chemotherapy. Your physician will

Complete blood count (CBC)

test performed on a blood sample; the number of red cells, white cells, and platelets in the sample is determined.

Red blood cells

blood cells responsible for transferring oxygen from the lungs to the tissues.

White blood cells

blood cells responsible for fighting infections.

Platelets

blood cells responsible for blood clotting and wound healing.

monitor your child's blood count to anticipate low values following chemotherapy, and may order a transfusion of red blood cells or platelets to prevent side effects such as feeling tired. (White blood cells are not transfused except under very special circumstances.)

Red blood cells (RBCs) carry oxygen throughout the body. When RBC values fall too low, children will complain of fatigue. This condition is called **anemia**. The CBC measures RBCs in many ways, but the simplest measure is either **hemoglobin** (measure of hemoglobin within the RBC) or **hematocrit** (percent of the blood that is made up of RBCs). One or both measures can be tracked. The need for transfusion is variable and depends on many factors. However, a transfusion may be considered when the hemoglobin falls below 8 g/dL or the hematocrit drops below 25%.

Platelets function to control bleeding (along with other coagulation proteins in the plasma). Your child may experience easy bruising and bleeding from the nose or mouth when platelets are low. The risk of bleeding increases when levels drop below 20,000. The platelet count is followed closely after your child receives chemotherapy. Aspirin and similar medications interfere with platelet function, causing the blood to take longer to clot, so such medications should be avoided.

White blood cells (WBCs) fight infection, and different types of WBCs are programmed to fight different types of infection. By far the most important infection-fighting cell is the **neutrophil** (also called a "PMN"). Your physician will follow the number of neutrophils carefully as the risk of infection rises with

Anemia

a condition resulting from low counts of red blood cells in blood.

Hemoglobin

a protein carried by red blood cells that picks up oxygen in the lungs. The hemoglobin measurement assesses the amount of this protein in the red blood cells.

Hematocrit

a measurement of the percent of the blood made up of red blood cells.

Neutrophil

a type of white blood cell; major defense against bacteria and fungal organisms.

neutrophil counts below 500. This is called the absolute neutrophil count or ANC (see Question 51 to learn how to determine ANC).

Leukemia, which starts in the bone marrow, can completely replace normal blood cells with cancerous cells so that blood counts are extremely low. Moreover, leukemia cells may be detected in the bloodstream and therefore can be detected by a CBC.

You should familiarize yourself with the normal values for the CBC (Table 1), and ask a member of the medical team to go over the numbers with you.

14. What is a biopsy?

When a tumor is suspected, often a small piece of the tissue is removed surgically and this sample is processed in a laboratory for diagnosis. This procedure is called a **biopsy**. A pathologist, a doctor who specializes in tumor diagnoses, examines the tumor under the microscope. In addition, the pathology lab runs a battery of tests to classify the cancer more precisely. It may take many days to run these tests, and it is crucial to be absolutely certain that the particular subtype of the tumor be defined precisely, since treatment is different for each cancer, even those within the same class of tumors. These tests often consist of determining the types of proteins that are expressed on the surface of cancer cells, because the proteins show which type of tissue the cancer originated from. They are the clues for the pathologist to figure out the exact type of abnormal cells. For example, certain proteins are expressed by muscle cells, and if these proteins are found to be expressed by the tumor, it is likely to be a

Biopsy

A surgical procedure that involves obtaining a tissue specimen from the body for laboratory testing to determine a more precise diagnosis.

Table 1. Values that might appear on the CBC report

Test	Units	Normal Values	Comments
White blood cell count[a]	$\times 10^3/mm^3$	4.5–17.5	Total infection fighting cells
Red blood cell count	$\times 10^6/mm^3$	3.9–5.3	RBCs, anemia
Hemoglobin[a]	g/dL	11.5–15.5	Measure of RBCs, anemia
Hematocrit[a]	%	35–47	Measure of RBCs, anemia
MCV	fL	76–90	Size of RBCs, increased when taking chemotherapy
MCH	pg	24–30	Amount of hemoglobin in RBC
MCHC	g/dL RBC	33–34	Concentration of hemoglobin/RBC
RDW	%	8–14	High in iron deficiency
Platelet	$\times 10^3/mm^3$	159–350	Measure of platelets, bleeding
Mean platelet volume	fL	7.4–10.4	Young platelets are a larger size

(continued)

Table 1. Values that might appear on the CBC report (continued)

Test	Units	Normal Values	Comments
Neutrophils (PMNs)	×10³/mm³	1.5–8.5	Most important infection-fighting cells in the body
	(%)	(30–70)	
Bands	%	0–5	Young neutrophils
Lymphocytes	×10³/mm³	1.0–4.5	Infection-fighting cells, but not as important as neutrophils (PMNs)
	%	20–70	
Monocytes	%	4–7	Sign of recovering WBCs, good infection-fighting cells
Eosinophils	%	2–4	Increased with allergy or infection
Basophils	%	0–3	Increased with allergy

Normal values vary according to age and gender, so all of the values listed are approximate. Abbreviations are: CBC, complete blood count; MCH, mean corpuscular hemoglobin; MCHC, mean corpuscular hemoglobin concentration; MCV, mean corpuscular volume; RBC, red blood cell; RDW, red cell distribution width; WBC, white blood cell.

rhabdomyosarcoma. If bone-forming proteins are present in the tumor, then it is an osteosarcoma.

As noted in Part One, cancers occur due to acquired mistakes or mutations in the DNA of a cell. Some of these mutations are quite specific, and tests can be performed to screen the cancer to determine the type of mutation, and therefore the tumor type. Each cancer is best treated with a unique combination of chemotherapy. Once the diagnosis is established, effective treatment can be planned.

15. What are tumor markers?

Tumor markers refer to certain substances, made by cancer cells, that can be detected in the blood or urine. These substances therefore serve as a "marker" to track the cancer. As such, these **tumor markers** can indicate whether the cancer is dying, because the number (level) of tumor markers decrease with treatment, or whether the cancer has become resistant to treatment or has recurred (because the levels increase). A few common tumor markers are shown in Table 2.

In addition to the detection of substances secreted by cancer cells, very new laboratory tests are available that

Tumor markers

certain substances made by cancer cells that can be detected in the blood or urine.

Table 2.   Common tumor markers.

Type of Cancer	Tumor Marker	Detected In
Liver tumor	α-fetoprotein (AFP)	blood
Germ cell tumor	AFP and β-human chorionic gonadotropin (β-HCG)	blood
Neuroblastoma	Catecholomines (HVA and VMA)	urine

allow physicians to track extremely small numbers of cancer cells in the body. These tests rely on a special technique called **polymerase chain reaction (PCR)**, which can detect one tumor cell within a background of more than a million normal cells. At present, only a few types of cancers can be tracked this way, but leukemia is among those that can be followed.

Polymerase chain reaction (PCR)

a laboratory technique that can detect one tumor cell within a background of more than a million normal cells.

16. What is staging?

The extent of involvement by the primary tumor (the location where the cancer first developed) determines the cancer's **stage**. Stages may differ between tumor types. One of the most important distinctions is whether the tumor is "local" (centralized to a single spot) or has spread (metastasized) to other parts of the body. A series of tests will be done to determine whether the tumor has metastasized. Many of these tests will be radiographic procedures to look at the lungs, sites in the abdomen and pelvis, and bones. Often a sample of bone marrow and spinal fluid will be taken to see if tumor cells have spread to these sites.

Stage

a method of describing how far a cancer has progressed; a higher stage number means greater progression.

No universal staging system exists for all solid tumors. Many cancers are staged depending on whether the tumor can be completely removed at diagnosis. For example, Stage I usually means the tumor has been completely removed at the time of the biopsy. When the sample is examined under the microscope, no tumor cells can be seen at the margins of the resected specimen (i.e., the surgeon removed the tumor cells and extra section of cells around it so that no tumor cells were left behind). If the surgeon removes the tumor but small numbers of tumor cells can be seen microscopically in the "margin" portion of the cells that were removed, then the tumor qualifies as Stage II. If the surgeon is unable to remove the tumor completely, it is called Stage III; and if the tumor has spread to other sites in the body, it is a Stage IV tumor. For other tumors, the site of the initial involvement (e.g., head and neck vs. a particular organ or extremity) as well as the number of sites involved are key parts of the staging system (see Table 3 for lymphoma).

Leukemias are not staged like solid tumors because they are blood cancers, and therefore tumor cells are seen throughout the body at diagnosis.

Obviously, cure rates are higher for lower stages. However, even Stage IV diagnoses may be cured, but these require more therapy. The goal of treatment for all types of childhood cancer is to provide enough therapy that the cancer is completely eradicated and the child is cured while avoiding unnecessary treatment since the side effects of cancer therapy can be quite serious.

Table 3. Lymphoma Staging

Stage	Description
Stage I	Disease is limited to one site.
Stage II	Disease is present on two adjacent sites on one side of the diaphragm (a structure that divides the chest from the abdomen).
Stage III	Disease is present on different sides of the diaphragm (although large lymphomas may be classified as stage III even if they occur on one side of the diaphragm).
Stage IV	Disease is present in bone marrow and spinal fluid.

Other factors are considered in addition to the stage when planning therapy. They include the particular subtype of cancer (for example, alveolar vs. embryonal rhabdomyosarcoma) or what it looks like under the microscope (e.g., favorable vs. unfavorable Wilms tumor or neuroblastoma). You should ask your physician to tell you the stage of your child's cancer and how this affects treatment options.

17. What is a bone marrow aspirate?

The bone marrow is the spongy, internal space of bones where new blood cells are produced on a daily basis. Leukemia starts in the bone marrow, and many solid tumors, including lymphoma, neuroblastoma, and other tumor types, can spread or metastasize to the bone marrow. Your child's physician may check the bone marrow often to determine whether tumor cells might be present. A **bone marrow aspirate** is performed by taking a small needle and inserting it directly into the marrow (Figure 3). A liquid sample of bone marrow is with-

Bone marrow aspirate

collection of a sample of bone marrow using a small needle to determine whether tumor cells are present.

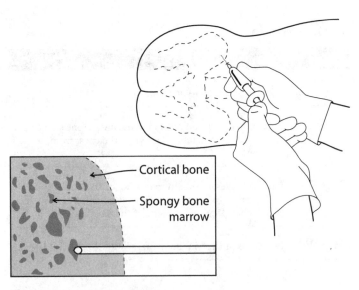

Cortical bone

Spongy bone marrow

Figure 3.   Bone marrow aspirate.

drawn and can be examined under the microscope to determine whether cancer cells are present. This specification helps a physician with the diagnosis, and the results can be reported very quickly. This procedure is usually performed while your child is under sedation in a monitored setting. There is typically some mild discomfort at the site of the procedure, but this discomfort is well managed with pain medicine.

"As far as helping parents explain the information to their children, I usually tell children that the blood is like a report card of the body that the doctors use... the bone marrow aspirate is the best way to find out how/what their body is doing. Also, in general, parents can focus their explanations to young children around the senses: what they will see, feel, hear, and smell is the most important information prior to procedures."

—Senior child-life specialist

18. What is a bone marrow biopsy?

A **bone marrow biopsy** is a procedure in which the very small solid "core" of the bone marrow, containing both the spongy scaffold and bone marrow itself, is withdrawn. A bone marrow biopsy may detect clumps of tumor cells that may not be seen in a bone marrow aspirate. Sometimes the aspirate may be dilute, and the biopsy usually provides a better representation of how many bone marrow cells reside within the spongy space. The procedure is completed with a small needle and does not require a surgical incision. The needle stick is somewhat painful, so these procedures are usually done with sedation, especially in young children. There are no known long-term side effects from the procedure.

Bone marrow biopsy

procedure involving needle insertion to remove the solid core of bone marrow.

Diagnosis

19. What is a spinal tap?

Some tumors originate in the brain and spinal cord, and some cancers like leukemia and lymphoma may spread (metastasize) there. The brain and spinal cord (called the **central nervous system** or CNS) are bathed in a thin reservoir of liquid called spinal fluid. A **spinal tap** or lumbar puncture (LP) is a procedure in which a sample of spinal fluid is extracted. Doctors can then view this fluid under a microscope to determine the presence of tumor cells. The actual procedure is simple. A small needle is inserted into the lower back, in between the vertebrae. This area is below the spinal cord, so there is very minimal danger of any injury. The spinal fluid sample can be taken, and medicine, if needed, can be given through the same needle during the spinal tap procedure. Spinal fluid is generated in your body constantly, so there is no danger of depleting spinal fluid, and the amount withdrawn is small compared to the total volume. An anesthetic cream may be applied to the area ahead of time to decrease any pain from the needle stick or, more commonly, the child may receive medicine intravenously to put them into a deep sleep (called **conscious sedation**). Some adolescents and young adults opt to undergo the "tap" with no sedation.

20. What is an MRI, and how does it work?

Magnetic resonance imaging (MRI) is a relatively new technique that allows the inside of the body to be scanned without using x-rays. One of the most important advances in medicine has been the development of sophisticated techniques to image the human body.

Central nervous system (CNS)

the brain and spinal cord.

Spinal tap / lumbar puncture

procedure in which a sample of spinal fluid is extracted in order to determine the presence of tumor cells.

Conscious sedation

light sedation; a "deep sleep" caused by intravenous medication.

Magnetic resonance imaging (MRI)

a scanning technique using radiofrequency pulses to affect the magnetic field alignment of hydrogen atoms, allowing doctors to view inside the body without using x-rays.

Detailed pictures of the internal structures of the body are now possible. These pictures allow physicians to get a detailed image of tumors as well as the ability to detect small metastases elsewhere.

MRI uses radio frequency pulses to capture black-and-white images that reflect the characteristic of the tissue being examined. Intravenous contrast medium (a liquid) can also be used with the MRI to assess whether blood vessels in the vicinity of the tumor are "leaky" (important in brain tumors) and whether tumor cells are dying. MRIs can be very sensitive in detecting abnormal changes in "soft tissues" such as the brain, spinal cord, and muscles.

21. What is a CT scan, and how does it work?

Computed tomography (CT), another imaging technique, uses an x-ray source that rotates 360° around the patient. The x-rays are detected by a series of devices rather than conventional radiographic film, and then a computer reconstructs thousands of images. With a CT, contrast medium (a liquid) is given intravenously to highlight blood vessels and to optimally image the liver, spleen, and kidneys. Oral contrast is given to distinguish bowel loops from masses or tumors in the abdomen and pelvis.

Computed tomography (CT)

a scanning technique that utilizes an x-ray source that rotates 360 degrees around the patient; can reveal many soft tissue structures not shown by conventional radiography.

22. When is an MRI requested, and when is a CT utilized?

MRI is now the method of choice to image the brain and spinal cord, while CT is still used to evaluate tumors in the chest, abdomen, and pelvis. MRI is also the best method to visualize musculoskeletal tumors. It must be emphasized that minor changes that occur normally in the organs/body, such as a resolving lung infection or post-surgical changes, can now be seen by these images. On occasion these resolving, reparative processes might be confused with metastasis or tumor growth. In such cases, the physician might order a follow-up study sooner to resolve these questions. These "false alarms" occur relatively commonly and can be a great source of frustration and anxiety for parents and children.

23. What is a PET scan?

Positron emission tomography (PET) is one of the latest and most exciting tools to assess whether masses are made up of viable tumor cells or scar tissue. PET is now the optimal way to determine early whether a cancer is responding to treatment. Currently, there is no conclusive way for a physician to know whether an identified mass is composed of dead cancer cells and scar tissue or of living tumor cells. One way to help distinguish among these possibilities is to inject a radioactive tracer that is taken up by an organ, and then track the metabolism of the tracer. In the most common application, labeled glucose or sugar is injected intravenously and the fate of the radioactive tracer can be detected. Glucose is an energy source, and metabolically active structures like cancers (and some normal organs like heart muscle) take up the glucose tracer.

A significant number of cancer cells die before a change in the physical dimension of a tumor can be seen. The quicker the cancer dies, the more likely it is that the treatment is effective and the patient will be cured. The PET scan can help oncologists differentiate

Positron emission tomography (PET)

a research imaging technique using short-lived radioactive substances that picks up active tumor tissue but does not measure its size; can assess whether masses are made up of viable tumor cells or scar tissues.

between the cells they see in the image. For many cancers like lymphoma, reassessment using a PET scan shortly after the start of therapy is becoming standard practice. PET scans are now replacing older nuclear medicine studies such as gallium and thallium scans. PET scans do not give as detailed a three-dimensional image as a CT scan, so the two techniques complement one another. However, new machines have recently been developed that combine the two techniques.

24. What is ultrasound?

Ultrasound uses high-frequency sound waves to image internal structures such as the heart (called an echocardiogram) and kidneys. Sound waves are applied through a **transducer** that is applied gently to the body surface. The transducer also receives sound waves as they are reflected off the surface of an internal organ. An advantage of ultrasound is that no radiation is used. Ultrasound is an effective technique to determine whether an abdominal mass originates from the kidney (Wilms tumor), adrenal gland (neuroblastoma), or liver (hepatoblastoma or hepatocellular carcinoma). Moreover, it is used frequently to assess the dynamic, blood-pumping action of the heart. Subtle differences in function due to the side effects of chemotherapy can be detected early using ultrasound.

Ultrasound

Type of imaging technique using high-frequency sound waves; useful in diagnosis but not particularly accurate in assessment of tumor response.

Transducer

Device that converts one type of energy to another.

PART THREE

Treatment Options

What is my child's prognosis?

What is remission?

What does "cure" mean, and is there a risk of relapse?

More ...

Cancer treatment has improved dramatically over the past three decades, and progress has been especially rapid in the treatment of childhood cancers. Treatment can involve surgery, radiation therapy, and chemotherapy. In some cases all three types of treatment are used, and in others only one type may be needed. Within childhood cancer treatment, the goal of therapy is to tailor treatment so that the chances for cure can be maximized while short- and long-term side effects of treatment are minimized.

25. What is my child's prognosis?

Your child's prognosis—the forecast of the probable course of the disease and its outcome—will differ depending on the type of cancer that is diagnosed and the stage at which it is diagnosed. Statistics offered in Figure 4 are a guideline and in no way indicate your child's individual chance for cure or survival.

In our experience, the fear of death is the first concern that all newly diagnosed patients and their families confront. Death and/or an inability to cure are potential realities for any child facing a life-threatening illness. However, the *majority* of children with cancer are cured. Confidence in your chosen oncologist, your education about the disease and its treatment, and a positive attitude will help you and your child throughout the treatment process.

*The **majority** of children with cancer are cured.*

26. What is remission?

A patient is considered to be in **remission** when there are no visible signs of the cancer by physical examination, laboratory tests, and/or radiographic tests (i.e., x-ray, CT scans, PET scans, MRIs, etc.). For some

Remission

complete or partial disappearance of the signs and symptoms of a disease in response to treatment.

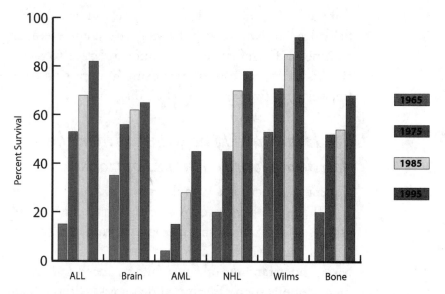

Figure 4 Five-year survival rates for childhood cancers. Figures generated from End Results Group at the National Cancer Institute and the Surveillance, Epidemiology and End Results (SEER) program.

tumors, remission might be achieved after one month of chemotherapy (in the case of leukemia) or after a combination of chemotherapy, surgery, and/or radiation. However, remission does not indicate cure since small numbers of cancer cells, too small to be detected, can still be present. For this reason, treatment is continued even after remission is first achieved.

27. What does "cure" mean, and is there a risk of relapse?

By definition, cure means that there is no evidence of disease, and the chances of it coming back are extremely low. Yet, cure is a nebulous term since there is always a chance that the cancer may return in the future. The risk of relapse is greatest while the patient is on a treatment regimen or shortly following the

"Cure" means that there is no evidence of disease, and the chances of it coming back are extremely low.

completion of therapy. The risk of relapse is substantially less at two years following the completion of treatment. Therefore, it is common practice to say a child is "cured" of cancer after being in remission continuously for five years after their diagnosis.

28. How quickly do we need to make a decision about treatment options?

Cancer treatment is a complex process. As a parent, it is difficult to have a complete understanding of all aspects of the illness and therapy within the first few days of diagnosis. However, it is critical that you have a basic understanding of your child's cancer and treatment options soon after initial diagnosis. Although an appropriate diagnostic evaluation and subsequent treatment decision need to be done quickly, it is unusual that therapy needs to be started immediately. For almost all childhood cancers, waiting a few days to a week to make a decision about treatment will not interfere with the chances for cure. However, there are circumstances that do require immediate attention and the initiation of treatment. Yet emergencies should not interfere with effective communication and, once resolved, you need not feel obliged to continue treatment until all issues are addressed to your satisfaction. Ongoing education is imperative, and time most likely will allow you to become more comfortable and secure with the treatment.

Waiting a few days to a week to make a decision about treatment will not interfere with the chances for cure.

"We found comfort in learning that most treatment is standardized. We had already spent 7 weeks running around to different doctors before he was even diagnosed. We just wanted to start on the road to cure."

—Parent of a child diagnosed with leukemia

29. When is surgery required?

One of the best ways to eradicate cancer is to surgically remove it completely at diagnosis. Surgery is used to remove "solid" tumors (see Question 14), not those that are "liquid" tumors (see Question 10). Removing only part of the tumor usually does not lead to a better outcome, so the timing of when (or if) to undergo surgery is critical. When the surgeon is confident that the whole tumor can be removed along with a surrounding "margin" of normal tissue (to be certain no tumor cells are left behind), surgery might be performed at diagnosis. If the tumor is too large, if it involves critical normal organs adjacent to the tumor, or if it has spread to other parts of the body, the surgeon may elect to perform a biopsy first and then start chemotherapy (see Question 29). The goal of the chemotherapy would be to shrink the mass. A "second look" surgery might then be done at a time when complete surgical removal is possible. The other value of a second surgery is that the pathologist can determine microscopically how many tumor cells have been killed by the initial application of chemotherapy. Those tumors that shrink the most in response to treatment and have a maximum amount of tumor cells killed by the chemo- or radiation therapy before surgery are associated with the best prognosis.

30. What is chemotherapy?

Chemotherapy refers to a large group of medications that are used in treating cancer. The type and dose of chemotherapy drugs depend on the cancer being treated; some drugs work optimally on certain cancers and not others. These medications can be given into the vein, taken by mouth, and/or inserted into the spinal fluid. Cancer is best treated with a combination of chemotherapeutic drugs, since some cancer cells

Chemotherapy
Drug treatment utilizing chemicals that have a toxic effect on the disease; some are designed to limit cell growth while other types kill specific cells.

within a tumor may be resistant to a single drug. Moreover, drug combinations may be given on a rotating schedule, again to avoid tumor cells from gaining resistance to treatment (see Table 4).

Most chemotherapies work by interfering with the way cells divide. Since cancer cells grow abnormally, they are generally more sensitive to the effects of chemotherapy as compared to normal cells. Chemotherapy, however, can damage normal cells. This factor accounts for many of the well-known side effects of treatment. Table 4 includes a list of commonly used chemotherapy drugs and some of their side effects. You should ask for a complete list of the drugs and their side effects that your child will receive. The complete list includes rare but sometimes scary side effects, and a complete discussion of these issues with your oncologist should take place before therapy is started.

"Another way to explain to your child may be to say, 'Chemotherapy is the very special medicine that fights very hard to make the cancer [boo-boo, etc.] go away'".

—Senior Child Life Specialist

---

31. Can my child receive vaccinations while on chemotherapy?

Live viral vaccines like the oral polio and MMR (measles, mumps, rubella) vaccines should never be given to children receiving chemotherapy, since even the weakened virus may cause an infection in a patient with poor immune status. Brothers and sisters of children with cancer should receive the killed polio vaccine (e.g., IPV [inactivated polio virus], the one given by a "shot" instead of by mouth). Fortunately, the killed or inacti-

Table 4.   Common chemotherapy drugs

Drug	How It Works	How It Is Given	Side Effects	
			Common	Infrequent/Rare
Asparaginase	Prevents protein synthesis *Used for:* Leukemia Lymphoma	IM	Allergic reactions	Pancreatitis Bleeding and/or blood clots
Bleomycin	Inhibits DNA *Used for:* Hodgkins disease Solid tumors	SQ, IM, IV		Lung fibrosis
Busulfan	Inhibits DNA *Used for:* Solid tumors BMT	PO	Nausea Low blood counts	Infertility Second cancers
CCNU/lomustine	Inhibits RNA/DNA *Used for:* Brain tumors	PO	Nausea Low blood counts	Liver/lung damage

(continued)

Treatment Options

59

Table 4.   Common chemotherapy drugs (continued)

Drug	How It Works	How It Is Given	Side Effects	
			Common	Infrequent/Rare
Cisplatin	Inhibits DNA *Used for:* Solid tumors	IV	Nausea Kidney damage Low magnesium	Hearing loss
Carboplatin	Inhibits DNA *Used for:* Solid tumors	IV	Nausea/vomiting Low blood counts	Nerve damage
Cyclophophamide (Cytoxan)	Inhibits DNA *Used for:* Leukemias, Lymphomas Solid tumors	IV, PO	Nausea/vomiting Low blood counts	Bladder irritation Electrolyte disturbance (SIADH) Infertility Second cancers
Cytarabine (AraC)	Inhibits DNA *Used for:* Leukemias Lymphomas	IV, IT, SQ	Low blood counts Mouth sores Eye irritation	Liver disease Difficulty with balance

(continued)

Table 4. Common chemotherapy drugs (continued)

Drug	How It Works	How It Is Given	Side Effects	
			Common	**Infrequent/Rare**
Dactinomycin (Actinomycin D)	Inhibits RNA synthesis *Used for:* Wilms tumor Rhabdomyosarcoma	IV	Nausea/vomiting Skin ulceration if drug leaks out of blood vessel	Mouth sores Liver damage Radiation recall
Daunorubicin (Daunomycin)	Interferes with DNA synthesis *Used for:* Leukemias Lymphomas	IV	Nausea/vomiting Low blood counts Mouth sores Skin ulceration if drug leaks out of blood vessel	Heart damage Second tumors
Dexamethasone (Decadron)	Initiates cell death *Used for:* Leukemias Lymphomas	PO, IV	Increased appetite Irritability/personality change Muscle weakness GI irritation High blood pressure	Diabetes Irritation of pancreas Bone problems
Docetaxel (Taxotere®)	Inhibits cell division *Used for:* Solid tumors	IV	Low blood counts	Lung damage

(continued)

Treatment Options

Table 4.   Common chemotherapy drugs (continued)

Drug	How It Works	How It Is Given	Side Effects Common	Side Effects Infrequent/Rare
Doxorubicin (Adriamycin)	Inhibits DNA synthesis *Used for:* Leukemias Lymphomas Solid tumors	IV	Low blood counts Nausea/vomiting Pink color to urine	Heart damage Second tumors
Etoposide (VP-16)	Damages DNA *Used for:* Leukemias Lymphomas Solid tumors	IV, PO	Nausea/vomiting Low blood counts	Allergy Low blood pressure Second tumors
Fludarabine	Inhibits DNA synthesis *Used for:* Leukemias	IV	Nausea/vomiting Low blood counts	Nerve damage
5-Fluorouracil	Interferes with NA/RNA *Used for:* Solid tumors	IV, PO	Nausea/vomiting Low blood counts	Diarrhea

(continued)

Table 4. Common chemotherapy drugs (continued)

Drug	How It Works	How It Is Given	Side Effects Common	Side Effects Infrequent/Rare
Gemcitabine	Blocks cell division *Used for:* Solid tumors	IV	Nausea/vomiting Low blood counts Liver damage	Fatigue Mouth sores
Idarubicin	Inhibits DNA/RNA synthesis *Used for:* Leukemias Lymphomas	IV	Nausea/vomiting Low blood counts Pink color to urine	Mouth sores Heart damage
Ifosfamide	Inhibits DNA *Used for:* Leukemia Lymphomas Solid tumors	IV	Nausea/vomiting Low blood counts	Irritation of bladder Infertility Second tumors Kidney damage
Imatinib mesylate (Gleevec)	Inhibits specific proteins (called Abl and PDGF) involved in growth signaling *Used for:* CML/ALL	PO	Weight gain Fluid retention Low blood counts	Liver damage Rash Fever

(continued)

Treatment Options

63

Table 4. Common chemotherapy drugs (continued)

Drug	How It Works	How It Is Given	Side Effects		
			Common	**Infrequent/Rare**	
Irinotecan	DNA damage *Used for:* Solid tumors	IV	Diarrhea Nausea/vomiting Low blood counts	Liver damage	
Melphalan	DNA damage *Used for:* Solid tumors BMT	IV	Nausea/vomiting Low blood counts Skin ulceration if leaks from blood vessel Mouth sores	Infertility Low blood counts	
6-Mercaptopurine	Inhibits DNA synthesis *Used for:* ALL	PO, IV *Do not take with milk.* *Give at bedtime and/or on an empty stomach.*	Low blood counts Decreased appetite	Liver damage	
Methotrexate	Inhibits DNA synthesis *Used for:* ALL Solid tumors	PO, IV, IM, IT *Give at bedtime and/or on an empty stomach.*	Low blood counts Mouth sores Liver damage	Brain damage Learning disability	

(continued)

Table 4. Common chemotherapy drugs (continued)

Drug	How It Works	How It Is Given	Side Effects	
			Common	**Infrequent/Rare**
Mitoxantrone	Damages DNA *Used for:* AML	IV	Nausea/vomiting Low blood counts Skin ulceration if leaks Mouth sores Urine blue/green	Heart damage Second tumors
Paclitaxel (Taxol)	Inhibits cell division *Used for:* Solid tumors	IV	Low blood counts	Numbness Allergy
Prednisone	Initiates cell death *Used for:* Leukemias Lymphomas	PO	Increased appetite Personality changes Stomach irritation	Diabetes Demineralization/damage to bone
Procarbazine	Inhibits DNA and RNA synthesis	PO *Do not take with alcohol, cheese, yogurt or chocolate.*	Nausea/vomiting Headache	Second cancer

(continued)

Treatment Options

65

Table 4. Common chemotherapy drugs (continued)

Drug	How It Works	How It Is Given	Side Effects Common	Side Effects Infrequent/Rare
Rituximab	Monoclonal antibody that leads to loss of B-cells *Used for:* B-leukemias Lymphomas	IV	Fevers/chills Allergic reactions	
Temozolomide (Temodar™)	DNA damage *Used for:* Brain tumors	PO	Low blood counts Nausea/vomiting	Nerve/brain damage Second cancers
6-thioguanine	Damages DNA *Used for:* leukemia	PO *Do not take with milk.* *Give at bedtime and/or on* *an empty stomach.*	Low blood counts Nausea/vomiting	Liver damage
Thiotepa	Damages DNA *Used for:* BMT	IV	Nausea/vomiting Low blood counts Mouth sores	Infertility
Topotecan	Damages DNA *Used for:* Solid tumors	IV, IT	Nausea/vomiting Low blood counts	Liver damage Flu-like symptoms

(continued)

Table 4. Common chemotherapy drugs (continued)

Drug	How It Works	How It Is Given	Side Effects	
			Common	**Infrequent/Rare**
Tretinoin (ATRA)	Induces differentiation *Used for:* APML	PO Take with fatty foods	Headaches Fever Fluid retention High white blood count	Bleeding Increased pressure in the brain
Vinblastine	Prevents cell division *Used for:* Hodgkin disease Histiocytosis	IV	Ulceration if leaks out of blood vessel Low blood counts Constipation Decreased reflexes	Nerve damage Allergy
Vincristine	Prevents cell division *Used for:* ALL	IV	Ulceration if leaks out of blood vessel Low blood counts Constipation Decreased reflexes	Nerve damage

Abbreviations are: ALL, acute lymphocytic leukemia; BMT, bone marrow transplant; CML, chronic myelogenous leukemia; DNA, deoxyribonucleic acid; GI, gastrointestinal; IM, intramuscular; IT, intrathecal (into the spinal fluid); IV, intravenous; PDGF, platelet-derived growth factor; PO, by mouth; RNA, ribonucleic acid; SIADH, syndrome of inappropriate secretion of antidiuretic hormone; SQ, subcutaneous.

vated polio vaccine is now recommended routinely for all children. Siblings can receive the MMR vaccine without any danger to a family member being treated for cancer.

The only exception to the live virus rule is the varicella, or chicken pox, vaccine, which has been given to children with cancer who are receiving treatment. It is common practice to check the immunity to chicken pox at diagnosis. If your child has not been vaccinated or immunity is very low, she/he may be susceptible to the chicken pox virus. This can be a serious infection in someone receiving chemotherapy. It is essential that you notify your doctor if your child is exposed to someone with chicken pox or someone who breaks out with it a few days after contact with your child. Injection of varicella zoster immune globulin (VZIG) right after exposure may protect a child from getting the disease entirely or may limit the intensity of the disease.

Killed or inactivated virus vaccines such as the DTaP (vaccinates against diphtheria and pertussis) and Hib (vaccinates against a serious disease caused by bacteria) can be given to children undergoing chemotherapy, although the vaccines may be not as effective. Many oncologists wait until the child is off therapy for three to six months to complete the vaccination schedule. Patients who have undergone a bone marrow transplant receive complete re-vaccination starting at 12 months post-transplant.

The flu or influenza vaccine may be recommended for patients on treatment especially when a heavy flu season is anticipated. However, the new live viral vaccine is not recommended. Household family members should also receive the vaccine to help minimize the chances of getting the flu. Both household members and patients should receive the standard, inactive vaccine.

32. How is chemotherapy administered? What is the difference between a broviac central line and a medi-port?

One of the biggest breakthroughs in the delivery of effective cancer therapy is the use of **indwelling central venous catheters**. These devices are very similar to the common intravenous (IV) lines used to give fluids and medicines. However, these lines are tunneled underneath the skin (usually in the chest) to anchor them, and they enter a major blood vessel near the heart. These central venous catheters are placed surgically or by a radiologist.

A percutaneous indwelling catheter (PIC) is inserted like a regular IV, but the tubing is threaded centrally into a major blood vessel. PIC lines are easier to place but can be useed only for a few months. A PIC is shown in Figure 5.

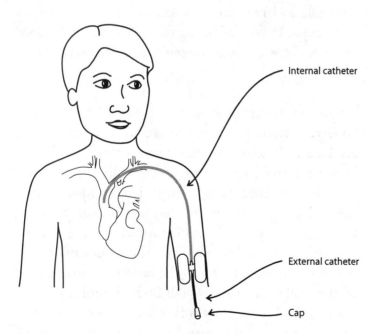

Figure 5   A percutaneous indwelling catheter (PIC).

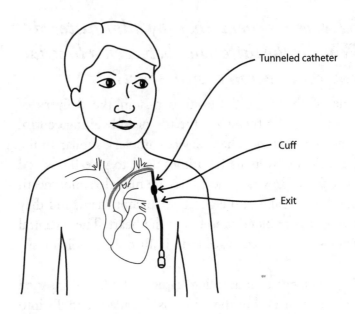

Figure 6   A broviac catheter.

Broviac

a type of central venous catheter; a specific type of tubing that is placed through the chest wall into a large blood vessel.

A **broviac** type line (Figure 6) exits the skin surface and can be accessed directly. A portion of the line is always accessible and no further "needle pokes" are needed to gain access. Instead of lasting days, they can be in place for years if needed. They are removed at the end of treatment.

There are many pros and cons associated with a broviac. Advantages of a broviac are that no pain is involved with access and that two (or three) additional lines can merge into the single central line, thus allowing multiple medicines, transfusions, and/or nutritional supplements to be delivered simultaneously. Furthermore, some chemotherapy can cause surface burns if the medicine leaks into the tissues under the skin surface. Since access to the broviac occurs outside of the body, the risk of a leak is diminished. The downside of broviac lines is that bathing is complicated because of the need to prevent a significant amount of water from getting underneath the dressing. Moreover, swimming is exceedingly difficult, if not impossible, without danger of infection. Broviac lines require more frequent access (about two to three times per week) with solutions to keep them open, that is, prevent them from clotting if they are not in active use.

In contrast, a **medi-port device** (Figure 7) uses a line leading to a reservoir that is located underneath the skin. When access is needed, a needle is placed through the skin into the reservoir. The benefit of a medi-port line is that it is located underneath the skin. The medi-port is not visible through most clothing and tends to attract less attention from others. For teenagers and children, this may allay their having additional concerns about a negative body image, feeling "different" from others, and feeling self-conscious, all of which are commonly associated with a cancer diagnosis for teens and children. The lack of external access eliminates concerns

Treatment Options

Medi-port

a type of central venous catheter; device that utilizes a line leading to a reservoir that is located underneath the skin.

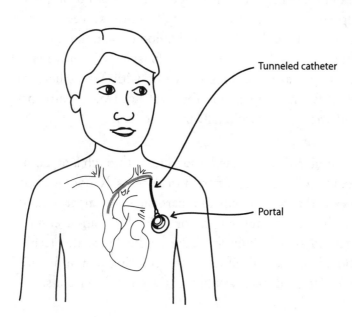

Tunneled catheter

Portal

Figure 7   A medi-port.

associated with bathing and swimming. In addition, medi-ports only have to be accessed once a month to prevent clotting when not in use.

Negative aspects include greater danger of infiltrating the underlying tissues with potentially harmful drugs, and the discomfort felt when the needle is inserted through the skin into the reservoir. Medi-ports also leave a slightly larger surgical scar than broviac lines after they are removed. Some chemotherapies may lend themselves better to specific catheter options. Speak to your doctor about your options.

33. What is a clinical trial, and how will our child's treatment be affected if we decide to participate?

Clinical trial

a research study, with patient participation, developed with hopes of improving medical care.

A **clinical trial** is a research study, with voluntary patient participation, developed with hopes of improving medical/cancer care. Despite great successes over the past three decades in childhood cancer, not all children are cured. In an effort to constantly improve cure rates, pediatric oncologists work with researchers to identify and implement the best available treatments and attempt to continually improve them.

Clinical trials are generally conducted through a randomized trial comparing different treatments. Randomization means that assignment to a particular treatment is done by chance, like flipping a coin. Randomization ensures that no bias is built into the study. Thus, the results should be scientifically accurate, ensuring that an identically designed study would find the same data results.

Subjects who enter a study are divided into different groups, called "arms," according to the particular study design. It is important to remember that in most instances, each arm of a randomized trial includes an already established treatment for a particular cancer. The test drug(s) is then built into that existing plan. In almost all cases the treatment plans are quite similar but differ in a small, but potentially meaningful way. For example, one plan may introduce a new drug, and perhaps another plan may administer an existing drug at a different dose or schedule.

You do not have to participate in a clinical trial, and if you decline your child should receive the standard treatment that has been established. Moreover, if you decide initially to participate, you have the option of withdrawing from the trial at any point. Your physician will keep you informed about the results of clinical trials, and you should feel free to ask about any new findings related to the care of your child's cancer.

Newer cancer-fighting medications are being developed each year, and some of these "experimental" medications may be available in tightly controlled clinical trials. These drugs are often tested in adults first before they are used in children. A phase I clinical trial determines the safe dose of a new drug—it is not designed to find out whether the drug actually works against a given cancer. A phase II trial uses the safe dose (determined in the phase I trial) and concludes if it is effective against a range of cancers. Treatment of recurrent or unresponsive disease is not often straightforward, so you should spend time investigating all options.

34. What is a protocol?

Fortunately, an appropriate treatment plan for all childhood cancers has been established. Years of careful study conducted by nationwide groups who review and compile findings and feedback from clinical trials (like the Children's Oncology Group [COG]) have led to the development of actual treatment plans, or protocols. A **protocol** is a written document that explains the background for a given approach to treating cancer. It includes specific instructions about staging and the types as well as the doses and schedules of chemotherapy. For clarity, treatment is described in courses and cycles, which distinguish different phases of treatment. Many protocols are part of a clinical trial.

Protocol

a formula, a treatment "recipe."

> *"Parents may find it helpful to ask for a copy of their protocol and fill it out as they go along. Then they can anticipate upcoming treatment and time commitments."*
>
> —Pediatric oncology nurse

35. How do I keep track of my child's treatment?

Effective cancer therapy involves the use of many different medications that are delivered in a particular sequence. In an effort to ensure that the treatment schedule is followed precisely, a series of **roadmaps** are used as part of a protocol. This roadmap documents which drugs are given at different points in treatment (the roadmaps are outlined within the protocol). Each phase of treatment has its own roadmap: a printed sheet showing the day that each medication is due and the dose of the particular drug. You can think of these roadmaps as a calendar of treatment. Your oncologist

Roadmap

a calendar of treatment(s).

and his/her staff will review your roadmap with you and your child. It is helpful to remember that the roadmap serves as a guide, and your doctor will adjust the protocol as necessary. Feel free to ask questions, stay abreast of the guide, and prepare accordingly.

"Always read your roadmap to help prepare yourself mentally for what is coming up next. But don't obsess about it."

—Parent of a child diagnosed with leukemia

36. What is radiation therapy?

Radiation therapy is a very useful treatment for many tumors in children. Optimally, one of the best ways to cure cancer is to remove it surgically. However, in many cases complete removal is impossible without damaging important normal organs or because surgery would leave an unacceptable cosmetic result. The value of radiation is that normal tissue (such as blood vessels and solid organs) can be maintained relatively unharmed within the radiation field while the cancerous cells are exposed to the radiation.

Radiation is delivered in fractions over many days to avoid damage to normal tissues. Different tumors vary in their sensitivity to radiation therapy, and therefore the total dose (and duration of treatment) varies considerably. For example, some brain tumors and sarcomas require high doses of radiation, whereas leukemias and lymphomas are more sensitive to radiation and therefore require less treatment.

The most common radiation technique uses an external beam to deliver an energy field composed of electrons or x-rays (photons) directly to the tumor. The resulting field directly damages tumor cells and leads to their destruction. Since radiation is delivered in a beam, it is useful for specific-area treatment only (with the exception of total body irradiation that is used in bone marrow transplantation). New techniques can pinpoint the radiation dose to a very small area (**gamma knife**) or configure the field to better align treatment with tumor margins while avoiding any surrounding uninvolved areas (e.g., **intensity-modulated radiation therapy** [IMRT]).

"For children and teens (and parents) I think it is important that they understand that radiation does not hurt, and it is generally for a few minutes each time. (Kids hear radiation therapy and they think Star Trek!) If children are not going to be sedated, they should be prepared for the "seat belt" that will remind them to lie still. In addition, even though mom and dad are not in the room, they are right outside and can see the child the entire time. The kids have a very important job: to lie still. The RT table/machine is very big, so they should be prepared for that as well."

—Senior Child Life Therapist

37. What is a bone marrow transplant?

The field of bone marrow transplantation has evolved rapidly in recent years. A **bone marrow transplant** is a procedure that allows a patient to have increased doses of chemotherapy in the hopes of improving chances for a cure. In some cases a particular cancer might be partially responsive to treatment; that is, some tumor cells may die but other residual or resistant cells cannot be eradicated completely. It is believed that if the dose of

---

Gamma knife radiation

a technique that can pinpoint the radiation dose to a very small area.

Intensity-modulated radiation therapy (IMRT)

a technique that can configure the field to better align treatment with tumor margins while avoiding any surrounding uninvolved areas.

Bone marrow transplant

procedure in which a section of bone marrow is taken from one person and transplanted into another; used to replace bone marrow that has been damaged or diseased.

chemotherapy could be increased, then the remaining more-resistant cells would also succumb to treatment.

Many tumors are treated first with conventional chemotherapy to significantly shrink the number of tumor cells in the body. At a certain point in the treatment, if the tumor is highly resistant, very high doses of chemotherapy, and in some cases total body irradiation, are applied to eradicate resistant residual tumor cells. The normal bone marrow is extremely sensitive to the very high doses of treatment. In fact, the marrow may never recover after the high doses. To "rescue" the patient from these toxic side effects, normal bone marrow is transfused back into the patient following high-dose chemotherapy.

The normal bone marrow cells quickly join with the patient's bone marrow, and brand new bone marrow begins to grow. It takes two to three weeks or longer for new blood cells to reappear in the blood circulation. During this time the patient is dependent on transfusions and at great risk for infections. The patient is generally isolated during this time.

38. What is the difference between allogeneic and autologous transplantation?

In bone marrow transplants (BMT) the reinfused bone marrow cells may come from many different sources, and this choice depends on the cancer being treated. BMT is the treatment of choice for acute myelogenous leukemia (AML) and relapsed acute lymphocytic leukemia (ALL). Since these are blood system cancers (liquid tumors), it is usually impractical to use the patients own bone marrow because it is likely to be contaminated with residual leukemia cells. In this case the bone marrow comes from an outside donor, who often is a brother or sister, or perhaps a closely matched parent. This is called an **allogeneic transplantation**.

A BMT also can be considered for certain solid tumors, including neuroblastoma and some brain tumors. In these cases, the patient's own bone marrow might be collected early in treatment and then reinfused after high-dose therapy. This is called **autologous transplantation**. An autologous BMT may also be considered in cases of relapsed lymphoma. Even though this is considered a cancer of the blood/lymphatic system, the patient's own bone marrow is less likely to be involved, so "autotransplants" are also considered in this circumstance.

39. Who can be a bone marrow donor?

The donor marrow must be matched to the recipient's **human lymphocyte antigen (HLA)** type in order for a BMT to be successful. HLA molecules are present on the cells of the body, and they allow the immune system to recognize and destroy foreign germs. The immune system would reject transfused bone marrow cells unless the HLA type was closely matched. When undergoing an autotransplant, HLA matching is not a concern since the patient's own bone marrow is reinfused.

However, in an allogeneic transplant the best option is an HLA-matched brother or sister. Since each child inherits a portion of their HLA type from each parent,

---

Allogeneic transplantation

a bone marrow transplant in which the marrow used for the procedure is supplied by someone else, usually a HLA-matched relative.

Autologous transplantation

a procedure in which a patient's own healthy marrow is collected prior to treatment and then reinfused after treatment.

Human lymphocyte antigen (HLA)

molecules in the body that allow the immune system to recognize and destroy cells that don't belong.

most parents are "half matches." However, some HLA types are extremely prevalent, so it is possible that parents might share certain HLA types.

More recently, a large number of individuals have volunteered to be BMT donors and their HLA type is stored in a computer. A **matched-unrelated transplant** ("MUD" transplant) is where the donor marrow comes from an unrelated individual. Since this individual is not related to the recipient, there are additional concerns as compared to a matched-related donor (see Question 41). Your oncologist can help you to determine whether a transplant is possible and who would be an appropriate donor.

Matched-unrelated donor transplant

a transplant procedure in which the donor marrow comes from an unrelated individual who nonetheless is matched to the patient's HLA type.

40. How is bone marrow harvested?

Bone marrow is harvested by inserting a small needle into the pelvic bone and withdrawing the liquid bone marrow into syringes. The needle needs to be inserted many times to obtain enough bone marrow. The bone marrow is eventually combined into a single blood transfusion bag and stored for later use. The donor is anesthetized during the procedure and may feel some temporary discomfort afterwards. The amount of bone marrow collected is usually small relative to the total bone marrow in the body, and the donor's bone marrow quickly replaces the lost cells. However, the donor may experience some fatigue during this time.

41. What is graft versus host disease?

One of the concerns associated with bone marrow transplant is **graft versus host disease**, or GVHD. Unless donor stem cells come from the patient's own blood or an identical twin, the donor's stem cells are

Graft vs host disease (GVHD)

a common and serious complication of bone marrow transplantation where there is a reaction of donated bone marrow against a patient's own tissue.

not identically matched to the recipient's HLA type (see Question 42). In this circumstance two conditions might arise. The recipient's (that is, the patient's) body could recognize the donor stem cells as foreign and reject the transplant (e.g., **graft rejection**). However, in most cases high-dose chemotherapy has weakened the recipient's immune system to the extent that rejection does not occur. On the other hand, the donor stem cells could recognize the recipient's organs as foreign, which leads to damage of the gut, skin, liver, and other organs. This condition is called graft vs. host disease.

Graft rejection

a situation in which the donated marrow is recognized as foreign and destroyed by the immune system.

It is not stem cells themselves that are causing the damage, but small numbers of T-cells present in the donated stem cells. These T-cells could be removed from the donation, but current research is focused specifically on understanding which subset of T-cells causes GVHD, since some T-cells may actually be useful in attacking any residual tumor left after the high-dose therapy.

42. What are stem cells?

In recent years, scientists have been able to identify and purify stem cells that are present in the background of normal bone marrow blood cells. Stem cells are very young blood cells that are capable of reestablishing a fully functional bone marrow when reinfused into the patient. Stem cells exist in much lower numbers compared to the types of blood cells that function every day to carry oxygen (red blood cells), stop bleeding (platelets), and fight infection (white blood cells). Stem cells are able to develop into all of these cells and might be thought of as "seeds" that germinate the bone marrow. They are also plentiful in the umbilical cord blood of newborn infants.

Currently it is common for stem cells to be harvested from the bloodstream directly, thereby avoiding harvesting the bone marrow itself. Blood is withdrawn from the donor and circulates in a machine that isolates the cell fraction containing the stem cells, and finally returns the rest of the blood to the donor.

43. We have heard about using cord blood for a stem cell transplant. Can we use our newborn child's cord blood? How do we store the cord blood?

Cord blood is rich in blood stem cells and can be used after high-dose chemotherapy instead of bone marrow. Graft vs. host disease appears to be less of a concern when cord blood is used. Therefore, "mismatched" cord blood has been used when a suitable matched product is not available from an adult or older child. However, cord blood transplants seem to have a higher failure rate compared to stem cells from older individuals, so some transplant centers will only use cord blood when other options are not possible.

It is important to note that any child has only a 25% chance of being fully matched with a brother or sister (see Question 39). Thus, the idea to conceive a child because a parent is motivated by the chances of securing a donor for another son or daughter who is a candidate for transplant is not ideal, for many reasons. With the development of cord blood/bone marrow

Cord blood
blood harvested from the umbilicus at birth and stored against the possibility of a need for transplant.

Treatment Options

"banks," there is a very good chance that a suitable unrelated donor might be identified.

Cord blood can be harvested from the umbilical cord after the baby has been delivered. The blood cells can be frozen for use in the future. However, this can be done only in select hospitals, so it is important to bring this issue to the attention of your obstetrician early in the course of your pregnancy if you are interested in pursuing this option.

The growth of cord blood banks have led to the idea that perhaps cord blood should be stored on every baby, just in case that child should ever need a bone marrow transplant in the future. There are many problems with adapting such a universal approach routinely. First, the chance of any individual needing a transplant is extremely rare and by itself does not justify a universal banking approach. Second, for some types of leukemia, abnormal cells can be detected at birth, so the marrow would not be appropriate to use in the future when dealing with leukemia.

44. What happens if the cancer doesn't respond to therapy or comes back?

Almost all cancers respond initially to treatment, and most go away completely. However, individual cases may not respond or the tumor may come back after a remission was achieved. Subsequent treatment options will then depend on the tumor type and timing of the reoccurrence.

Almost all cancers respond initially to treatment, and most go away completely.

The treatment that is initially prescribed is based on vast clinical experience accumulated over the past two to three decades in treating that particular tumor. However, no two cases are exactly alike, and response to treatment cannot be predicted accurately in all cases. If the tumor fails to respond to the initial treatment, therapy will be switched to a chemotherapy combination that has shown promise in select cases. This combination may not be designated "front line" therapy because the response rate overall is not as good as the combination tried initially.

If the tumor comes back once remission has been achieved, somewhat different approaches are used depending on the timing of reoccurrence. Tumors that reoccur are generally less responsive than tumors at initial diagnosis. If the patient has been off treatment for some time, then there is a reasonable chance that some of the same drugs used the first time around may still be effective. If the child suffers a reoccurrence while on therapy, the chances of that being the case are less likely. In either case, new drugs are introduced since the tumor has not developed a resistance to them. Some of the same drugs may be used to treat a relapse, but they may be more effective if given at higher doses.

45. What happens when treatment is complete?

Although the final day of therapy is anticipated with great joy, it can be an unsettling event for parents and patients. It is normal and appropriate to be filled with mixed emotions at this critical stage in the treatment process. The perception may be that the chemotherapy is suppressing the cancer and that it will come back when therapy is no longer applied. Yet, in fact, therapy is predetermined to be extended to an interval beyond which most cancers are cured. This provides a safety margin. Clinical trials have determined that additional extension of therapy beyond the standard time provides no advantage to cure and may actually lead to serious side effects.

In addition, transitions can be difficult for everyone, and it is important to acknowledge and lend credence to all of the emotions that you experience as your child completes therapy. The changes can be unsettling. The sights, sounds, and faces are familiar and comforting. It can be challenging to break the clinic/hospital routine and return to your old schedule. The experience of diagnosis and subsequent treatment will forever change your reality. You will inevitably experience a new "normal" as you attempt to integrate the experiences into your life.

The experience of diagnosis and subsequent treatment will forever change your reality.

In terms of medical management, at the end of therapy a series of tests are done again to confirm that no signs of cancer are detected. These tests may consist of laboratory work including tumor markers if possible, imaging tests like MRI or CT scans (solid tumors), and bone marrow and spinal fluid examinations for leukemia. All treatment is stopped, not tapered, and the patient is followed on a regular basis in the doctor's office. The exact schedule differs among tumor types, but can be every one to three months for the first year and less frequently thereafter, since the risk of recurrence diminishes significantly with time. The same tests used to diagnose and follow the cancer's response to treatment will be repeated in the follow-up period. Scans may be repeated every three months for the first year, every four to six months during year 2, and less frequently afterwards. At some point, the need for surveillance testing stops completely when the risk of cancer reoccurrence is very low.

In addition to tests that determine any signs of cancer reoccurrence, some tests will be done to look for possible side effects of treatment. These tests would include cardiac echocardiograms (ECHOs) and possibly other tests for patients who have received the drugs adriamycin or daunomycin. Levels of certain hormones, such as thyroid or growth hormone, will be assayed for patients who have received irradiation to the brain and/or thyroid. These tests may also be indicated in cases where surgery has been performed near hormone-secreting centers in the brain.

Overall growth and development require constant assessment as well. The overwhelming majority of patients achieve normal heights (although they might be slightly shorter because of cancer therapy). Also, although most children do well in school, some children who received therapy directed to the central nervous system, especially at a young age, may experience neuro-developmental side effects. These may include a delay in being able to accomplish some mental or physical tasks relative to other children of their same age bracket. Periodic assessment, including standardized testing, may be indicated in high-risk patients. A major goal of long-term follow-up is to detect potential side effects early so that intervention techniques to minimize their impact can be established.

PART FOUR

Side Effects and Complications of Treatment

Are new medicines available that don't have the same side effects typically associated with conventional therapy?

What is considered an emergency for my child while on treatment?

What can we do to prevent side effects of treatment?

More ...

The treatment of childhood cancer has improved dramatically, but cancer treatment involves strong, potentially toxic therapies. Although the benefits of therapy outweigh the risks, the medical team will work to avoid or minimize these side effects.

46. Are new medicines available that don't have the same side effects typically associated with conventional therapy?

New drugs are being developed each year. Many of these agents are modifications of existing medications. However, increased understanding of cancer biology has led to the development of new classes of compounds that are now being integrated into conventional treatment.

Monoclonal antibodies are produced by a clone or fused hybrid cells, called a hybridoma, to establish cell lines that produce a particular antibody. These antibodies recognize specific proteins, and many have been engineered to recognize tumor cells. The antibody rituximab (sold under the trade name Rituxin®) has shown promise in adult lymphoma and is now being assessed for use with pediatric B-cell lymphoma. Similarly, the antibodies epratuzumab and alemtuzumab (CamPath®) are entering clinical trials in pediatric acute leukemia. Some of these antibodies have been coupled to drugs or toxins so that the antibody can deliver these agents directly to the tumor, where they destroy the tumor cells. Gemtuzumab (Myelotarg®) is one such example that is now being used to treat AML. Many antibodies were first developed for use in

Monoclonal antibodies

artificially produced antibodies that recognize specific proteins, allowing them to be aimed only at cancer cells.

leukemias and lymphomas, but antibodies directed for use with solid tumors are already in clinical trials, including those that are used to fight against the common tumor neuroblastoma.

The drug imatinib mesylate (Gleevec®) has ushered in a new generation of anti-cancer drugs: It represents the first example of molecular medicine. These therapies are targeted toward specific molecules (proteins) that occur on cancer cells. For example, there is an acquired mutation called the "Philadelphia chromosome" that drives cancer growth in chronic myelogenous leukemia (CML) and some cases of ALL. Laboratory studies have determined that the Philadelphia chromosome results in an overactive growth signal mediated by a particular protein that is only produced in the tumor and is not shared by normal cells. Scientists have now developed specific inhibitors that block this pathway, and imatinib is the first of these to undergo widespread use in patients. It is taken by mouth, has few side effects, and is extremely effective. Although it is unlikely to cure these cancers when used alone, it will improve cure rates when used in combination with other therapies.

Another promising new field is the area of **angiogenesis,** in which researchers seek to kill the tumor by attacking its blood supply. Cancers actually encourage the development of new blood vessels since tumor cells are highly dependent on a constant supply of nutrients carried in blood. Although early trials with "anti-angiogenic" agents were disappointing, a better understanding of the process and the development of more potent inhibitors of tumor blood supply will likely lead

Angiogenesis

ongoing research aimed at finding ways to prevent tumors from creating blood vessels, effectively starving the tumor.

to promising new directions for cancer therapy. The field of cancer biology is moving at a rapid pace, and you can keep abreast of developments by talking to your doctor or accessing some of the publications and Web sites recommended in the Appendix.

47. What is considered an emergency for my child while on treatment? Whom do we call in event of an emergency?

You should contact the doctor whenever you have concerns or questions. The treatment of cancer is a journey consisting of a partnership and communication between a family and their treating team. However, there are specific warning signs that should alert parents to contact their oncologist immediately:

There are specific warning signs that should alert parents to contact their oncologist immediately.

- Your child has a fever of 100.4°F or higher.
- Your child is vomiting or not eating.
- Your child is having difficulty or pain when going to the bathroom.
- Your child appears to have difficulty walking or has any change in speech, orientation to a person, place, or time.
- Your child is sleeping excessively.
- Your child is bleeding (e.g., from the gums or nose), has severe bruising, or has blood in the stool or urine.
- Your child is experiencing headaches or significant pain anywhere in the body.

If you are attempting to reach your doctor after clinic hours, you may connect by phone to an answering service, which can reach them by pager. Remember: Do not hesitate to contact your oncologist if you have any questions or concerns.

48. What can we do to prevent side effects of treatment?

It is impossible to prevent all side effects of therapy. Some common medications for side effects are listed in Table 5. If significant side effects occur, your child's doctor may adjust the dose of chemotherapy so that side effects are minimized or eliminated while maintaining an adequate level of anti-cancer treatment. Another common preventive strategy relies on the use of the drug Neupogen or G-CSF to minimize the degree of neutropenia (see Question 51) following treatment. Neupogen is a hormone that stimulates the production of normal white blood cells (neutrophils). G-CSF is normally made in the body. But by giving higher doses of the synthetic drug following chemotherapy, the blood count may be boosted more quickly, thereby minimizing the number of days at risk for infection.

It is impossible to prevent all side effects of therapy.

The amino acid called glutamine may be recommended to prevent mouth sores that can result from chemotherapy. Maintaining an adequate nutritional status is also very helpful in ensuring that the body recovers optimally from treatment effects. High dose vitamins have not been shown to provide a protective effect and in some cases may actually interfere with chemotherapy, or might cause side effects themselves. You should discuss any vitamin supplements with your doctor.

"It is important that patients be aware of the importance of hand-washing in general, but most importantly when neutropenic. Frequent hand-washing by the patient and all of the people with whom he or she comes in contact can help decrease chances for infection. Specific diet recommendations can also be helpful when attempting to minimize potential side effects of treatment."

—Pediatric oncology nurse

Table 5. Common medications used to treat the side effects of treatment

Drug	What It Is Used For	How It Is Given
Allopurinol	Prevents the build up of uric acid that can harm the kidneys	PO
Rasburicase	Breaks down uric acid that had already formed	IV
G-CSF (Neupogen)	Hormone that stimulates white blood cell production	SQ
Erythropoeitin (Procrit)	Hormone that stimulates red blood cell production	SQ
MESNA	Prevents damage to the bladder caused by cyclophosphamide or ifosfamide	IV, PO
Leucovorin	"Rescues" cells from the effects of methotrexate	IV, PO
Dexrazoxane (Zinecard®)	Prevents heart damage caused by adriamycin/daunomycin	IV
Bactrin or Septra	Antibiotic used to prevent pneumocystis pneumonia	PO
Pentamidine	Used to prevent pneumocystis pneumonia if patient cannot tolerate septra	IV, or by aerosol
Fluconazole	Antibiotic used to prevent/treat fungal infections	PO, IV

Abbreviations are: IV, by vein; PO, by mouth; SQ, injection underneath the skin.

49. What can we do to minimize the nausea and vomiting associated with chemotherapy?

Nausea and vomiting are some of the most troubling side effects of chemotherapy. Fortunately, for the most part they occur during the administration of the

Side Effects and Complications of Treatment

Table 6. Common anti-nausea medications

Drug	Comments
Granisetron (Kytril)	First-line therapy (PO, IV).
Ondansetron (Zofran)	First-line therapy (PO, IV).
Dexamethasone (Decadron)	Used in combination with first-line drugs. Should not be used long term or used as an anti-nausea agent in patients with leukemia/lymphoma (PO, IV).
Promethazine (Phenergan)	Used when nausea occurs despite first-line therapy. Can cause uncomfortable side effects, so often given with Benadryl (PO, IV).
Diphenhydramine (Benadryl)	Used in combination. Causes some sedation which may be the reason it helps with nausea (PO, IV).
Hydroxyzine (Vistaril)	An antihistamine like Benadryl (PO, IV).
Metoclopramide (Reglan)	Used when other medications fail. Can have side effects such as excessive nervousness and abnormal movements, so often is given with Benadryl. (PO, IV).
Lorazepam (Ativan)	Actually a sedative that can be quite effective in minimizing anticipatory nausea. Used in combination but is not given in conjunction with other medications that cause sedation (PO, IV).

Abbreviations are: IV, by vein; PO, by mouth.

chemotherapy and for one to two days afterwards. A number of measures and interventions can be used to minimize nausea and vomiting. The most effective combatant of nausea is the administration of anti-nausea medications before the chemotherapeutic drugs are started and regularly thereafter during the treatment even if nausea is not reported (see Table 6).

There are also interventions and useful techniques that do not involve administering medication. For example, distractions like television, movies, video games, or music are often helpful during administration of chemotherapy or medication. Elevating your child's head during or after chemotherapy may minimize nausea and vomiting as well. Odors can precipitate nausea, so it may help to leave food trays outside the room when your child is hospitalized and to avoid cooking odors in the home for one or two days after receiving particularly troubling drugs. Staying hydrated is more important than eating solid foods, so offer frequent sips of room-temperature, non-carbonated fluids. If your child is feeling well enough, serve "bland" foods like dry toast or crackers and avoid spicy foods. Interventions such as guided imagery and deep relaxation can be effective. Speak with the behavioral health team members to determine what could be helpful for your child. Finally, when traveling from the clinic or hospital, always be prepared for the possibility of vomiting; carry a basin, towels, and convenient pre-moistened (fragrance-free) wipes in the car.

50. What are the signs of infection?

One of the biggest side effects of cancer treatment is the risk of infection. Infections might be due to germs not commonly observed in healthy individuals, and they can be very serious. This increased risk of infection is caused by many factors. The most important risk factor is low white blood cells, specifically neutrophils (also called "polys" or "segs"), that commonly drop following treatment. In addition, a breakdown in normal barriers, such as irritation of the lining of the mouth and intestine (a condition called mucositis), is a common side effect of many anti-cancer agents. The presence of a foreign body such as an indwelling catheter (broviac or medi-port; see Question 32) in the bloodstream can serve as a focal point for bacteria, molds, and fungi to grow as well.

The most common indicator of infection is fever, so you should call your doctor immediately with the development of any fever (see Question 52). Although fever is the most common and reliable sign of infection, it might not be present if your child has very low blood counts or has been on steroids for long periods of time. In fact, steroids and low blood counts may mask many signs of infection; thus, it is important to be particularly vigilant during these periods. Other signs of infection may include redness or swelling over the site of the catheter or other parts of the body. Pain, especially if it is localized to one area, may indicate an underlying infection. In addition, a significant cough and diarrhea may indicate a respiratory and intestinal infection, respectively. Finally, a general change in behavior, such as serious fatigue that occurs suddenly, may indicate a generalized infection. You should call the medical team when any of these signs occur. When in doubt, call your doctor; he or she will instruct you about the next steps depending on your child's blood count at the time as well as other signs of infection.

When in doubt, call your doctor.

51. What is neutropenia, and how is it determined?

White blood cells (WBCs) are responsible for fighting infections in the body. Different types of WBCs perform different functions, and each type is uniquely suited to eradicating certain germs. Neutrophils (also called PMNs and "polys") are one major type of white blood cell, and these cells are a major defense against bacteria and fungal organisms. **Neutropenia** is a temporary decrease in the production of neutrophils and is a frequent side effect of chemotherapy. Typically, the neutrophil count will fall about one week or so after receiving chemotherapy, and it may take another two weeks for the body to make neutrophils again. Some forms of chemotherapy are more likely to be associated with neutropenia, and the medical team can predict when neutropenia might occur. During this time a patient may be quite susceptible to infections, so it is quite important to avoid people who might be sick (e.g., large crowds in contained spaces, such as a movie theater) and to call the doctor immediately if a fever develops.

Neutropenia

temporary compromised immune state in which white blood cells are decreased and risk of infection is great.

The neutrophil count, which would indicate if a patient was or was not neutropenic, can be determined through a routine blood draw. The lower the neutrophil level in the blood, the greater the chance of infection. The medical team relies on the absolute neutrophil count (ANC) to estimate the risk of infection. Once the ANC drops below 500/μL, the risk of infection increases substantially. The ANC is calculated by multiplying the WBC by the percent of neutrophils in the blood. For example, if the WBC is 4,700/μL and the laboratory technician determines that 60% of the WBCs are neutrophils, the ANC is 2820/μL (4,700 × 0.60 = 2820). It takes practice to do this calculation yourself (and it can be tricky since some labs report the WBC in different units). Most labs now calculate the ANC automatically, so it is best to ask for this value directly.

52. What is a fever?

Historically, fever is defined as a temperature greater than 38°C (100.4°F) rectally. However, due to the increased risk of infection, rectal temperatures should NEVER be taken in children with low blood counts. In general, most pediatricians recommend tympanic thermometers (e.g., in the ear) for routine assessment of temperature in all children. Surface temperatures such as ear and axillary (under the arm) are lower compared to temperatures recorded by mouth (oral). It is important to note that the body's core temperature undergoes a daily cycle (called circadian rhythm), with higher temperatures being recorded in the late afternoon and early evening.

Some centers use an arbitrary definition of fever as two temperatures of 100.3°F within an hour or a single temperature of 101°F to define fever. However, this definition varies between treatment centers somewhat, so you should consult your physician about his or her own standards concerning fever. If you are concerned that your child may be developing a fever, you should avoid giving your child medications such as acetaminophen (Tylenol) that may mask a fever and delay diagnosis. Because drugs like aspirin and ibuprofen (Motrin) interfere with platelet function, they should never be used when blood counts are low.

53. What are blood transfusions? How do we know if our child needs one?

A **transfusion** is an introduction of blood directly into the bloodstream. A transfusion consists of infusing "units" of red blood cells or platelets intravenously (IV)

Transfusion

an introduction of blood directly into the bloodstream.

to patients. A unit is defined as the amount of blood or platelets that is routinely harvested from a single donor. A red blood cell transfusion takes approximately four hours whereas platelets can be infused rapidly over fifteen minutes. The amount of blood or platelets required depends on the patient's size and the levels of blood counts prior to the transfusion.

Transfusions of red blood cells (RBCs) and platelets are frequently needed to be certain that these critical blood components are at a safe level. A low red blood count, called anemia, can be associated with fatigue, weakness, headache, and dizziness (especially when assuming a standing position after laying down or sitting). Low platelets are associated with an increased bleeding tendency. Signs of a low platelet count (called **thrombocytopenia**) include frequent nosebleeds that don't stop easily with pressure, bleeding from the gums, and bruising or **petechiae** (small pinpoint red spots that represent bleeding into the skin).

Thrombocytopenia
low platelet count.

Petechiae
small pinpoint red spots that represent bleeding into the skin.

54. What are the risks of a transfusion?

Transfusions provide critical support during periods of profoundly low blood counts. The medical team will order a transfusion only when the hemoglobin/hematocrit (two measures of red blood cell levels) and/or the platelet count are low. There are some immediate risks associated with transfusions. Reactions to transfusions include fevers (fairly common), hives and serious allergy (uncommon), and a blood incompatibility reaction (rare). Fevers may be minimized with Tylenol given before treatment, and mild allergic reactions can be prevented with medications like antihistamines (e.g., Benadryl). However, for more serious allergies, "washed" platelets might be given. The platelets are subjected to more stringent preparation before they are available to be transfused. Washing decreases platelet numbers, so it is not used routinely. In very rare cases, a blood incompatibility reaction can occur. This can result in blood pressure changes and serious kidney problems, so monitoring is always done during a transfusion.

One of the most concerning risks of a transfusion is the possibility of acquiring an infection. Fortunately, newer screening techniques have reduced the risk of acquiring an infection like hepatitis or the AIDS virus to 1 in 250,000 to 1 million.

55. Can we donate our blood for our child? Should family and friends donate blood for our child?

No transfusion is without risk but, as stated above, the risk of transmitting an infection now is quite rare. Scientific studies show that the risk of acquiring such an infection is no different between random volunteer blood products and donations from close friends or family members. Nonetheless, some parents prefer to use **donor-directed products**. A donor-directed product means that your blood donation is intended for a specific recipient. However, blood donors need to be matched for the right blood type, and this is especially true for red blood cells.

Donor-directed product

a blood donation made with the intention that the blood goes to a specific person.

It is important to consider a few issues regarding donation that need to be discussed thoroughly with your medical team. For example, if your child is a candidate for a bone marrow transplant, he or she should not receive blood products (e.g., platelets or red blood cells) from immediate family members. There is a risk that such a transfusion might lead to the development of immunity that could cause the patient to reject a bone marrow transplant that usually comes from a sibling or matched parent.

In some cases, cytomegalovirus negative ("CMV negative") products (e.g., from a donor who has never had a CMV infection) will be used exclusively for transfusions, and this might eliminate a healthy donor who would otherwise be an acceptable blood donor. CMV is a common virus that most people will acquire during their lifetime. The virus itself is usually associated with a mild infection, and although the virus might lie dormant in the body indefinitely, it rarely results in any significant illness. However, during periods of a profound decrease in immunity, it can cause a serious form of pneumonia (inflammation in the lungs). Therefore, potential exposure to the virus should be limited in patients undergoing very intensive chemotherapy.

56. Will our child be in pain?

It is reasonable to assume that your child may experience pain and/or discomfort at certain points in the course of treatment. Cancer, its treatment, and treatment side effects may be unpleasant and may create some difficult experiences for your child. However, most of the time he or she should be pain-free. Many steps are taken to ensure that your child endures a minimal amount of discomfort, and such strategies are discussed in this book. Skilled professionals at your treatment facility may be able to offer assistance.

"This strategy worked for us: we often remind our son that pain, discomfort, or other unpleasant side effects caused by the treatment are not forever. We try to provide any relief, even temporary, by addressing the problems individually and directly, like using a compress for itchy eyes."

—Mother of a patient diagnosed with leukemia

57. Is there anything that can be done to lessen our child's actual or anticipated pain and/or discomfort?

There are many interventions available to eliminate or lessen your child's discomfort and/or pain. A number of pharmacological and non-pharmacological interventions exist that can be used both in anticipation of the discomfort and to manage the actual pain associated with some procedures. For example, catheter placement helps eliminate the need for frequent peripheral line access. Thus, the child will ultimately undergo fewer needle sticks for blood tests and IV medication. Emla or Ela-Max crème, a topical anesthetic that is applied to the skin and left on for a fifteen or more minutes prior to needle access, can be used to numb the area where a needle is to be inserted. This cream can be obtained over-the-counter without a prescription.

Younger children are also sedated under an anesthesiologist's care during procedures that may cause severe discomfort, such as bone marrow biopsies and spinal taps. There are also many anti-nausea medications that are available to counteract the discomfort associated with the side effects of many types of chemotherapy. Anti-anxiety pills may also be provided by your doctor to be used very intermittently if anxiety levels seem to interfere with "normal" tolerance of treatment.

The child-life specialists at your child's treatment center are trained to provide specific interventions that aim to reduce fear, anxiety, and pain that children may have in response to anticipated or actual procedures. Depending on your child's developmental level, interventions provided may include medical play, familiarization play, guided imagery, relaxation breathing, and/or procedural accompaniment. Some of these interventions, such as **medical play** and familiarization play, are introduced and implemented in the playroom before procedures are performed to target a child's anticipatory anxiety or fear. By allowing children to familiarize themselves with real medical equipment and use it during play, children are given a sense of mastery and control over their environment, thereby decreasing the "scariness" associated with this new, confusing, or painful procedure.

Medical play

therapeutic technique used to help children understand their diagnosis and the medical environment.

Other interventions, such as **guided imagery** and **relaxation breathing**, are offered according to a child's age and are introduced before procedures to be utilized during procedures. The goal of these techniques is to equip children/teens with the tools they can use to counteract the physiological symptoms associated with pain or anxiety, including an increased heart rate, muscle tension, sweating, shivering, and vomiting. Whenever appropriate, child-life specialists are made available to accompany the patients through the procedure and guide their use of the techniques. At times, specialists will provide distraction through storytelling, magic tricks, or introduction of stimulating toys to redirect the child's focus from the procedure. Other

Guided imagery

psychological visualization technique used to counteract symptoms associated with pain and anxiety.

Relaxation breathing

a relaxation technique focused upon slow, controlled inhalations and exhalations.

trained professionals, such as music therapists, may offer interventions that address pain reduction and pain management. Psychology services may offer assistance with hypnosis, meditation, and/or exploration of feelings associated with pain.

"Pain management may be associated with an issue of control for your child. Let them be part of the solution."

— Mother of a patient diagnosed with a blood cancer

"It is important to note that the darker the skin, the longer that you need to wait to insure that the numbing agent is effective."

— Pediatric oncology nurse

58. What are the potential effects of radiation on the individual?

Early side effects of radiation treatment may include inflammation of the treated area such as a "sunburn" to the skin, irritation to lining of the oral cavity (mucositis, head and neck tumors), and diarrhea (abdominal tumors). Patients who get irradiation to the brain may experience fatigue. Late effects of radiation therapy depend on the dose applied. A big concern is the impact on long-term neurobehavioral functioning in children who have been treated for brain tumors. A formalized, neuropsychological evaluation/educational assessment is suggested before radiation begins and can be performed by a psychologist affiliated or recommended by your treatment clinic. This evaluation will assess the child's **cognition**, that is, activities associated with thinking, memory, and capacity to learn. Ascertaining your child's cognitive baseline before radiation begins can be useful

Cognition
thinking, memory, and capacity to learn.

as a future measure of any cognitive changes that result from radiation. Avoiding radiation in young infants is a common practice since young children under the age of 3 are particularly vulnerable to neurological impairment. Radiation to the brain can also affect hormone production, potentially resulting in a short stature and thyroid hormone deficiency. Fortunately, early diagnosis and replacement therapy can minimize these side effects. Finally, the most serious of all side effects is the development of a secondary cancer within the radiation site many years later. This is quite rare, and many such tumors can be treated effectively.

Early diagnosis and replacement therapy can minimize side effects.

59. What are the risks of all of the x-rays that our child will receive?

A small amount of radiation exposure occurs with procedures such as conventional x-rays, PET and other radionucleotide scans (bone scans, etc.), and CT scans (see Questions 19–22). Radiation has been shown to cause tumors, so there is always concern about unnecessary exposure. Yet, the dose used in these procedures is very small, and for practical purposes the risk of developing a second cancer is almost nonexistent compared to the benefit of these procedures. Regardless, specialists in pediatric oncology always work to limit the number of requested procedures. Moreover, facilities used to dealing with children will use lower doses compared to those used in adults. You can ask your doctor whether the radiology department at your hospital has significant experience with children and whether the facility has adapted new standards for children.

60. Will our child be sterile?

Certain forms of chemotherapy can make it more difficult or actually impossible for the child surviving cancer to conceive children in the future. Some treatment drugs are more likely to do this than others, and the risk of sterility increases depending on the total dose of medication administered. For example, drugs such as cyclophosphamide and ifosfamide, if given in high doses, can result in infertility. However, on many treatment plans the dose is low enough so that the risk is substantially diminished. Irradiation to the pelvic area and sexual organs carries a high risk of subsequent infertility. In some cases the ovaries may be positioned in such a way to avoid direct effects of the radiation treatment. You should discuss these issues with your child's physician to get an accurate assessment of your child's risk of infertility.

61. Can we bank our child's sperm or eggs?

If males are old enough, sperm can be banked before chemotherapy is initiated. Previous studies suggested that such samples have lower sperm counts before treatment even begins as a result of the disease. Yet, in many cases, technology has improved so that much fewer sperm are needed for successful in vitro fertilization in the future.

Unfortunately, egg harvesting is currently not available for children. However, new techniques are being developed to harvest eggs from females. While some of these techniques are still experimental and would only be available for adolescents or young adults, you should ask your doctor about their status.

62. Why will our child's hair fall out from treatment?

In most instances, your child's cancer will be treated with chemotherapy and/or radiation. As indicated earlier, chemotherapy is a strong combination of drugs that kill cancer cells and stop them from reproducing. Chemotherapy may not make the distinction between good and bad rapidly dividing cells, and subsequently attacks all cells that fall into this category, which include, for example, hair follicle cells. Not all chemotherapy drugs cause hair loss, so you should ask your child's physician about your child's treatment. In addition, hair loss may occur in some phases of the treatment and not others. This is particularly true of the treatment for ALL, where hair loss may occur during the first six to eight months of treatment, but hair will then grow back normally during the two to three years of maintenance therapy. The hair will grow back after chemotherapy is completed unless high-dose radiation was used to treat a brain or head/neck tumor. In this case the patient may be left with a permanently bald spot. However, the remaining hair, when long enough, can usually cover such an area.

Hair loss tends to be one of the more difficult side effects for children to accept. It is a constant physical reminder of their illness. Part Six will provide some suggestions and interventions to help your child deal with the realities of hair loss from chemotherapy.

63. Are there restrictions related to chemotherapy drugs?

Some chemotherapy agents have strict dietary guidelines. For example, while on an oral medication called procarbazine (generally used to treat solid tumors), large amounts of caffeine-containing foods or drinks, such as coffee, tea, colas, or chocolate, should be avoided. Certain foods, drinks, and drugs can cause high blood pressure if taken while receiving procarbazine therapy. These include certain cheeses, fava or broad beans, over-ripe fruit, meat, fish, or poultry that has been smoked or pickled. Avoid serving such items during the time your child is on procarbazine and for two weeks after he or she stops taking it.

If your child is receiving methotrexate, large amounts of folic acid need to be avoided, since folic acid can decrease the effectiveness of methotrexate. If high-dose methotrexate is being used, your physician will ask you to avoid sulfa compounds (examples are drugs such as sulbenzamide, sulfacytine, sulfadimethoxine, etc.) and other antibiotics that may interfere with the elimination of methotrexate. These medications can be resumed after the drug is no longer present in the body. Please ask your oncologist, nurse, and/or pharmacist for a complete list.

64. Are there eating restrictions during treatment?

Eating healthy and incorporating ample portions of all of the necessary food groups is always an important component of healthy living. Common-sense food preparations and adherence to basic Food and Drug Administration (FDA) guidelines, that is, eating well-cooked meat, should also be followed. Basic dietary restrictions will be recommended upon diagnosis, particularly when your child is neutropenic. There continues to be research on the interaction of diet and treatment, but at this time most oncologists follow these guidelines. Fried foods, raw foods (i.e., sushi) and those food items where cleanliness of the cooking source cannot be guaranteed (i.e., fast food restaurants) should be avoided when your child's blood counts are low. Fruits with skin that cannot be peeled, such as strawberries and raw vegetables, should also be avoided during periods of neutropenia. Avoid food from salad bars that are accessible to the public. Aged cheeses present the risk of increased bacteria, as do the above-mentioned foods. As with all of the recommendations in this book, consult with your treating physicians and staff regarding their eating restrictions/instructions.

65. Will our child's eating habits change during treatment?

Many factors account for decreased nutritional intake during therapy. At diagnosis, a larger number of tumor cells themselves produce substances called cytokines that result in profoundly decreased appetite as well as increased metabolic (energy) demands. In addition, your child's appetite and capacity to eat certain foods may be greatly affected during treatment.

Your child's taste buds, likes and dislikes for different foods, and appetite may change radically during treatment. Some of the therapies used to treat your child may make them sensitive to certain tastes and smells. In addition, the emotional aspects associated with cancer may affect your child's eating habits. When your child is nervous, afraid, or upset, changes in eating patterns are very common and normal. There can also be an increase in negative associations with foods as treatment progresses. For example, if your child became ill or nauseous after treatment and ate a certain food before or after getting ill, she/he may develop a dislike of that food.

Treatment and the subsequent side effects tend to affect your child's appetite, too. General weight loss and a decrease in appetite are common during cycles of chemotherapy. For example, during induction and a few other phases of therapy (in standard ALL treatment), nutrition might be compromised, but in general the treatment will not affect the appetite. In fact, steroid medications (e.g., prednisone or decadron), which are used in the therapy of ALL, actually cause an increase in appetite. In contrast, patients undergoing therapy for certain stage III and IV solid tumors and AML might need constant medical intervention to optimize weight gain at other points during therapy, especially if weight loss exceeds 10% of optimal weight for height.

Some treatments can result in painful mouth sores, which may interfere with your child's eating as well. It is important to be patient with your child's fluctuating weight and communicate with your child's physician. Be flexible regarding what your child wants to eat, and understand that there are medical reasons why they may become difficult to feed.

Be flexible regarding what your child wants to eat.

"We have our son drink a lot of water. We even play a game to see how much water he drinks in a day. We feel that the water is helping to cleanse his system, but we don't have to worry that it is going to interfere with treatment."

—Mother of a child diagnosed with leukemia

66. Are there any restrictions for oral hygiene during treatment?

Dental care is always important. Yet precautions need to be taken when your child is undergoing treatment and/or chemotherapy. You must check with your treating oncologist before any dental work, including a

Check with your treating oncologist before any dental work.

check-up, is performed. It is also necessary to inform your dentist that your child is currently being treated for cancer. If your child's blood count is low during the check-up, bleeding from his/her gums could result and the risk of infection may increase. Moreover, if a child has a central line, he/she might need a dose of antibiotics before a dental procedure to prevent infection. In general, while undergoing cancer treatment, teeth should be cared for with a soft toothbrush, which can help avoid irritating the gums. Rinse and care for your toothbrush to avoid unnecessary germs. Use dental floss with care. Be aware of the potential for mouth sores or irritated patches in the mouth. Always inform your oncologist of any concerns.

PART FIVE

Treatment Facilities and Healthcare Providers

What should we look for in an oncologist/clinic?

Can we get a second opinion?

How involved will our child's pediatrician be in treatment?

More ...

Cancer treatment requires many different specialists who focus on treating the patient and family, not just the disease. Treatment should consist of state-of-the-art medical therapy delivered in a warm and healing environment.

67. What should we look for in an oncologist/clinic?

Therapy for most childhood cancers has been clearly defined, and most childhood cancer centers are linked to common treatment approaches (for an extended description, visit the Children's Oncology Group Web site *www.childrensoncologygroup.org*). Therefore, there are few differences in treatment plans between individual pediatric oncologists. Access to optimal treatments most likely will not differ based on where you choose to undergo treatment. However, some pediatric oncologists may have expertise in a specific cancer and might be in a position to address unusual or challenging cases.

It is important to have confidence in your chosen oncologist and clinic staff. You may be presented with options in care, so knowing that you trust your doctor and his/her team will be of assistance in the process. Difference in personality, style, and approach may impact your comfort level. Do consider all of these variables when deciding about your treatment center.

Since you will be working very closely with your doctor, it is crucial that you are comfortable with his or her style and "bedside manner." Sometimes, for no particular reason, parents and a physician may not "connect," and it might be very appropriate to change to another primary doctor (see Question 67). As care may be provided by other physicians in your doctor's group, you should always feel assurance and comfort with the practice that you choose in general.

"All sorts of doctors and other medical specialists might be involved in a child's care: orthopedists, physical therapists, and dentists to name a few. It is important to work with a team who communicates well with each other."

—Mother of a child diagnosed with leukemia

"When we first found out our son had cancer we were devastated. Then we learned more about cancer and realized how experienced our oncologist and his staff were, and we felt more comfortable and relaxed."

—Father of an adolescent diagnosed with leukemia

---

68. Can we get a second opinion?

Most doctors encourage and welcome a second opinion. It is important that you and your family feel comfortable with your child's treating oncologist and suggested treatment protocol. Determining which clinic, doctor, and team are right for you is part of the process. Although conflicting opinions may cause stress, it may be a necessary step to take in determining what is best for your child. Consider all informed opinions, and take advantage of professional expertise with rare or challenging cases. In most cases, a second opinion will provide needed reassurance about treatment and does not indicate a lack of confidence in the initial physician or medical team.

Most doctors encourage and welcome a second opinion.

One way to introduce the topic of a second opinion to your current treating physician would be to express your gratitude for the care that your child has received and your comfort in the expertise of the physician and staff. Explain that your child's health is of such importance that you feel that a second opinion would provide additional reassurance on what is an almost impossible situation—the life-threatening illness that affects your child. Feel free to ask your physician about a recommendation as to where to seek another consultation. It is essential that accurate medical information be provided to the physician from whom you are seeking a second opinion, and communication between the physicians will facilitate the process. Do not be worried that feelings might be hurt. Experienced doctors and staff understand the desire to seek another opinion and will support you in your search. You can make this request at any point in the treatment plan. However, it is important to make an effort to consider why you are asking for a second opinion. A cancer diagnosis and subsequent treatment can be difficult to accept. Attempt to reconcile your need for a second opinion before you search and ask yourself whether you aren't just looking for a different response that you want to hear. Talking with mental health professionals, family, and friends may help you to discern your reasons for seeking alternative opinions.

"Getting a second opinion is also a way to understand more fully the disease and treatments, to collect information and understand what the process will entail. Not all treatment is the same for all cancers. Specialists or those more knowledgeable about a diagnosis may provide more insight."

—Mother of a young child diagnosed with ALL

69. How involved will our child's pediatrician be in treatment?

In many cases, a pediatrician will be the first to identify a potential diagnosis and suggest the family make an appointment with a specialist for further testing. Generally, when cancer is formally diagnosed, the oncologist will assume a majority of the patient's primary care. In an ideal situation, the pediatrician remains an essential member of the treatment team. However, once on therapy, given the complexity of care and the large number of potential issues related to therapy, all symptoms and concerns should be addressed to the treating oncologist first. If a family lives far from their treating facility and oncologist, special arrangements for more localized general care may be arranged. Encourage all physicians involved in your child's care, your pediatrician's office and your oncologist, to stay in contact and communicate with each other.

When cancer is diagnosed, the oncologist will assume a majority of the patient's primary care.

"Make sure that all of the doctors working with your child make an effort to communicate with each other."

—Mother of a young child diagnosed with ALL

70. Who are all these different doctors?

Many centers that treat childhood cancer offer specialized training for medical school graduates seeking training in general pediatrics and pediatric hematology/oncology. "Interns" are in the first year of their general pediatric training, while "residents" are in their second or third year. "Fellows" are physicians who have completed training in general pediatrics and are pursuing advanced training in a particular subspecialty like pediatric hematology/oncology. Although the number of doctors might seem bewildering at times, it ensures that your child and all medical concerns will receive maximum attention.

71. Who should we expect to encounter during my child's course of treatment?

The care of any child with cancer requires a large medical team with each member focused on some important part of the treatment plan. Optimally, one physician, usually a pediatric oncologist, will function as your child's primary doctor. It is her/his responsibility to coordinate all aspects of care: ordering certain diagnostic tests; planning treatment, including chemotherapy, surgery, and radiation if needed; and actually implementing the care plan. He or she is assisted by other members of the medical team, including radiologists, radiation therapists, surgeons, nurse practitioners, nurses, and pharmacists. You and your child will most likely meet many different medical practitioners as your treatment regimen progresses. Depending on the nature of your child's disease and treatment plan, various ancillary clinicians and departments may be involved in your child's care.

Cure involves more than just treating the medical condition itself, and this is especially true for treating childhood cancer. In addition to the team members mentioned above, social workers, child-life specialists, and psychologists focus on providing family-centered care that includes all physical and psychosocial dimensions of illness.

Your child will most likely interact with different types of medical technicians and other professionals when in the hospital as well. Your center may also have on-site financial counselors or billing department personnel who can help you navigate and understand your insurance coverage and billing. If this service does not exist at your center, ask to be referred to the hospital billing department or local advocacy groups. Your center may also have a parent education liaison, an experienced parent/caregiver of a cancer survivor who can help educate and support you and your family though the process. Every clinic or hospital is different, so be sure to understand the services and professionals available to you and your family.

72. What does a pediatric hematology/oncology social worker do?

A social worker should be available to your child and family depending on the facility where your child is undergoing treatment. In some facilities, a social worker will follow your child, whether inpatient or outpatient, while some facilities will have separate workers for each location. Find out the arrangement in your clinic or hospital. Services differ depending on needs and region of the country. Regardless, your social worker should act as a liaison between your family and outside agencies, as well as an advocate to address your needs and concerns. A social worker should be available for your concrete and clinical needs. Concrete needs include referrals for financial assistance from various cancer organizations, assistance with home care referrals, insurance concerns, providing educational material, and so forth. Clinical assistance includes supportive counseling with an emphasis on adjustment to illness. Some social workers also work with patients directly using a variety of interventions including art and play therapy, while other social workers run various support groups or can refer you for counseling in your community.

"Use, use, use (the) social work(er). No one has been more helpful to us. Use all available resources so you don't go crazy."

—Mother of a child diagnosed with leukemia

---

73. What and who is "Child Life," and how can it help?

Most pediatric clinics and/or hospitals that cater to children will have a Child Life Program. The Child Life Program at your hospital is designed to help meet the unique emotional and developmental needs of a child/teenager diagnosed with cancer or a blood disorder. The overall goal of the Child Life Program is to reduce the fear and anxiety associated with the medical environment, and to promote normal growth and development. The Child Life Specialist accomplishes this through a variety of therapeutic interventions, often centered on play.

Play is an important aspect of a child's development. Through play, a child can learn, express his or her fears, and master the environment. The Child Life Specialist uses play to help a child comprehend his or her diagnosis and to reestablish a sense of control over the environment. Child Life interventions include medical play, developmentally appropriate education, procedural accompaniment, self-expression through creative arts, the provision of essential life experiences (such as the promotion of peer interaction and the celebration of birthdays and holidays), and the assessment of a child's overall adjustment to illness/hospitalization.

Child Life Programs are often centered in playrooms. As the playroom is a safe haven for patients, medical procedures and discussions do not occur in the playroom. It is a place where children can have fun, and not feel threatened by the medical environment. One-on-one interventions take place in the playroom as well as group programs.

Child Life Programs may also provide additional therapeutic programs, including music therapy, recreation therapy, animal-assisted therapy (pet therapy), school re-entry programs, teen programs, and sibling support programs. Talk to your oncologist to determine whether these services are available to assist your child.

"Our family was in total shock at my son's diagnosis of leukemia at age two and a half. We were unsure how to make him feel at ease with the new reality. The Child Life program established at our hospital helped us navigate our new world. The trained professional recognized our bewildered looks. They greeted our entire family, friends, and visitors with genuine smiles and empathy. The Child Life team shared with us developmentally appropriate music, literature, and enrichment programs available to children of all ages."

–Mother of a child diagnosed with ALL

---

74. What if our child needs medical assistance at home?

Many medical procedures and treatments are performed in an inpatient or outpatient setting, monitored by healthcare professionals. However, there are instances when your child can receive interventions or medication distribution at home. Generally, medications not requiring constant monitoring or observation by a health professional can be administered at home (for example, medications such as Neupogen, antibiotics, and oral medication).

Home care must be approved by your oncologist and undergo an initial referral process for skilled nursing assistance. In addition, the patient and the family must be knowledgeable about their diagnosis and treatment, and the patient must be medically stable and have good intravenous access. The first dose of any medication and/or treatment should always be administered in a controlled medical setting to allow for the observation of reactions or intolerance.

75. How do we get home nursing care assistance?

After a patient has been approved to receive certain medications or procedures at home, a skilled nursing agency is generally contacted. In most hospital/clinic settings this nursing referral is initiated by a social worker, a nurse practitioner, or a discharge planner. Your insurance agency will be contacted and your home care benefits will be assessed. An in-network agency will then be contacted that services your area. The oncologist will provide the prescription requesting assistance to the home care agency and, depending on insurance coverage, may require the family to obtain supplies (e.g., medication and/or syringes). Extent and duration of assistance will vary with insurance plans. The ultimate goal for all home care agencies is to make a family proficient enough to administer certain medications (e.g., Neupogen) or perform dressing changes, without nursing assistance. Skills learned at home with the home care nurse will be reinforced during medical appointments.

76. What options are available if our child's cancer cannot be cured and palliative care is the only choice?

The obvious goal of all cancer treatment is to achieve a cure. In the event that your child's cancer cannot be cured, it is important to be aware that options for your child and your family do exist. Determining which option is best for your child is dependent on many variables. Where will your child be most comfortable? What are the wishes of your child? What are the emotional, physical, and financial abilities of your family? Medical limitations and available assistance will also likely play a role in your decision-making process.

Some families opt to remain in the hospital when no other viable treatment options are available. They gain comfort and security from the around-the-clock care available to their child. Medical personnel are easily accessible in the case of an emergency and to manage pain issues. The hospital environment helps to create a setting where family members can often avoid the dual role of being the caretaker and the parent. In the hospital, medical management is left to the professionals. Breaks and respite opportunities are more easily organized in the hospital. Families also gain access to support staff such as child life and social work.

If medically appropriate, families and patients may opt to remain at home. Families derive great support and comfort from a familiar environment. Children may voice that they prefer to be home, surrounded by their favorite things. Restrictions around visiting hours and visitors are eliminated. Comfortable sleeping arrangements for family members help them deal with the emotionally charged situation they confronted on a daily basis. A referral from your oncologist for home care will ensure that you receive personal attention from a scheduled visiting nurse while at home. Most medication and equipment can be made available to your child. At home, your child can avoid the constant intrusion of medical staff at all hours. The reduction in intrusion may allow for more quality interactions and conversations between you and your child. A referral may be made to **palliative care** (that is, care focused on alleviating the symptoms without curing the underlying disease). This referral will ensure that a social work team specializing in bereavement issues will come to your home to provide support as well.

Hospice programs, either at your home or in a facility, may be another option available. These programs focus on quality-of-life and pain control. The hospice facility creates a unique environment for your child and your family. The setting tends to be less "cold" and sterile than a hospital, but not as personal or intimate as your home. Professionals trained specifically in the needs and concerns associated with end of life are available there 24 hours a day.

All of these options are subject to possible financial and insurance limitations. Inquiries can be made on a case-by-case basis. Support services and available people should be utilized and involved in the process. Do not feel that you are making these critical decisions on your own. Any decision should be an informed one and is individually based on your situation.

Palliative care

care focused on alleviating the symptoms without curing the underlying disease.

Do not feel that you are making these critical decisions on your own.

PART SIX

Living and Coping with Cancer

How do we explain the diagnosis to our child?

Will our child's development or behavior be affected by treatment?

Can our child attend school during treatment?

More ...

A child's diagnosis of cancer affects many people and their lives. Understanding these effects and finding ways to integrate them into everyday living can help all those surviving with cancer. The focus of this section is on maintaining quality of life and placing the emphasis on *living* with cancer.

77. How do we explain the diagnosis to our child?

Explaining the diagnosis to your child will be difficult. Your own thoughts, feelings, and fears about the diagnosis will most likely be transferred to your child as you attempt to explain it and its implications. However, explanations in age-appropriate language are important to your child's overall integration of the diagnosis. Left to speculation and guesswork, your child will most likely assume the worst. Let your child know that this diagnosis is not their fault, that they have done nothing to cause it and could not have prevented it. Arming your child with appropriate information and education will help your child to feel some control over the situation.

Talk to your children. Listen to them.

Talk to your children. Listen to them. Find out what is going on in their heads. It is important that children know that they can ask questions and that they will be answered honestly. Although at times this may be difficult, it is almost always best to be truthful with your children. Kids have access to resources to find out information on their own, and accurate information can save them a lot of unnecessary worry. Depending on your child's level of communication or understanding, it may be helpful to utilize alternative mediums such as books, art, and play. Simple and direct explanations are most effective for younger children. Relate to them using examples and words that they can understand. For example, "you have a boo-boo in your blood and you need medicine to make you better," may be an appropriate explanation for a 2- to 3-year-old. For older children, it is helpful to use the correct terminology, as the child will frequently hear these terms and will need a clear understanding. Don't underestimate your child's intelligence or ability to understand. Adults are often surprised at how much children pick up and comprehend. Ask your child to repeat back the information you are explaining to gauge their level of comprehension.

If it is too difficult to address these questions at this time, the clinic where you are receiving treatment should have support staff—social worker, psychologist, Child Life Program staff, oncologist—available to help you with the words or to talk directly to your child. Be aware that everyone will have different expectations and understanding of the illness and its implications for themselves.

"Because our child was so young at diagnosis, we feel we will be answering this question throughout his lifetime, as he reaches different developmental stages. Yet, the one thing that is continual is our honesty. We try our best to always prepare him with what to expect from hospital procedures, effects of medicine, and routine clinic visits. It isn't always easy to share the news of the unpopular finger prick or access. We hope that the message is that he can rely on us for accurate information, which, in turn, appropriately validates his experience and feelings."

—Mother of a child diagnosed with leukemia

"I could go on and on here...children and teens do much better with procedures and treatment when equipped with information. Developmentally appropriate education can be delivered to your child in various mediums depending on your child's coping style."

—Child life specialist

78. Will our child's development or behavior be affected by treatment? What can be done to counteract those changes?

In general, children progress though various stages of development. There are age-appropriate behaviors and developmental tasks that comprise each stage (Table 7). Your child will be emotionally affected by a cancer diagnosis and its subsequent treatment. The extent and impact will differ depending on many variables, including your child's personality, the child's age, and the degree of support and intervention that your child receives during the process.

Your child will be emotionally affected by a cancer diagnosis.

Although not all children progress at the same rate, sometimes their individual rate of development changes upon diagnosis. The stress of having an illness may manifest when he/she is diagnosed, when in the hospital for an extended period, or over the course of a prolonged treatment. Your child may regress, behaving as if he/she were younger. For example, a child who has been toilet trained may start to wet the bed. Usually, this happens for a short time and the child will get "back on track" with minimal or no intervention. If you are unsure what is considered a "normal" reaction, or if you are concerned about your child's behavior, please consult a mental health practitioner at your clinic or hospital.

Not all children progress at the same rate.

Table 7. General Developmental Ages and Stages for Children

Age Range	Developmental Stage
Infant	
0–2 months	Vulnerable; primarily sleeps and eats, experiences the world through the body. Hears well. Can be calmed by soothing voice and cuddling.
2–6 months	Sleeps less; recognizes caregivers, makes eye contact; has a strong suck, active movement of extremities, and vigorous cry.
6–12 months	Verbal development starts; begins to roll over and then can sit alone; items are explored orally first; reaches for toys. Can be distracted or calmed with a pacifier or toy.
~1 year to 18 months	Begins to scoot or crawl, attempts to stand supported; later can walk and run. Clearly prefers caregivers and may experience stranger anxiety; is opinionated and illogical. Learns by trial and error. Labels things as "mine."
Toddler	
2–4 years	Egocentric ("the world revolves around me"); concrete thinker; narcissistic. Language development varies, but may understand what is being said while not being able to express well. Cannot distinguish between reality and fantasy. Can be distracted by play and favorite toys. Able to cope with being offered choices as it provides a sense of control; praise is important.
Primary School Age	
5–9	Able to express concerns (verbalizes about emotions); can understand cause-and-effect relationship; magical thinking/wishes; talkative and analytical. Can understand simple explanations about their treatment. As new skills are acquired, has a sense of accomplishment. Is developing autonomy (independence), and needs praise to affirm positive behaviors.
Latency	
9–12	Logical; socialization with peers is important; seeks more information to form an opinion. Has a sketchy concept of how the body functions, but wants to be an active participant in her/his own care. May be modest. Lacks common sense.
Adolescence	
12+	Problem solver; thinks abstractly. Struggles with independence, body image, sexuality, and peer pressure. May take risks and experiment with new behaviors, but does not like to feel "different" from peers. Shifts slowly from depending on family to friends for emotional support and social development.

Living and Coping with Cancer

Negative impacts such as stress and trauma can be minimized through many outlets. There are many resources available to assist your child in coping with and communicating about the experience.

Some facilities have staff that specializes in therapeutic interventions. Social workers, psychologists, and Child Life Program staff all utilize various means of expression (e.g., play, art, and talk therapy) depending on your child's developmental stage and level of engagement. Groups and/or family therapy may be a useful intervention to counter some of the feelings associated with this experience.

"Adjustment is hard, but always keep in mind that the priority is getting your child better. Everything else will take a back seat to this. (If you really feel that something is not right, your social worker can point you in the right direction)."

—Mother of a child diagnosed with a brain tumor

"Our child was two and a half when he was diagnosed with leukemia. It was hard to know what he was thinking and feeling because of his age. It was clear that he didn't like medicine administered by needles or the taste of some of his medicines. But that was obvious. The emotional effects and trauma were harder for us to identify. So we opted for play therapy to broaden and deepen his emotional vocabulary, to be able to discuss about hospitals in general, and his experiences specifically."

—Parent of a child diagnosed with leukemia

"Your child will do as well as you do. They take their cue from you. The bottom line is to let them know how much you love

them and that everything will be all right. A sense of security does wonders. Even if you don't feel it . . . give it to them."

—Mother of a child diagnosed with a brain tumor

79. How can we, as parents, help to minimize our child's behavioral changes associated with treatment?

Learning to follow rules is a normal part of growth and development for children. Discipline can be instrumental in assisting your child in learning to follow the rules. Yet, it may be difficult to discipline your sick child for a multitude of reasons.

It may be difficult to discipline your sick child.

Settings limits and restrictions can be very difficult for parents who are worried about their child's health and well-being. It can be very difficult to say "no" to your child when he or she is in pain and/or struggling with a diagnosis. However, when parents treat children differently than they are accustomed to being treated, kids sense that something has shifted. This shift is concerning for a child, who is already thrust into a rapidly changing new world. Structure and limit setting are normal parental functions and may provide reassurance to children who are experiencing a drastic change in their lives. When they feel as if there are no rules or structure, most kids feel out of control or overwhelmed. In general, it is ideal to set limits by encouraging positive behavior and cooperation, rather than threatening a child with punishment and consequences.

Yet, as indicated earlier, your child's behavior may change, and this change may not be within their control.

It may be a result of a child's medication, a current difficult emotional situation, or from fear or anger about an impending or current medical procedure. Parents need to be sensitive to the causes of the behavior change and do their best to not react when changes are not within the patient's control. Recognizing the enormous task of balancing your own feelings, concerns, and fears with those of your child can be difficult. Please don't forget that there are skilled mental health professionals prepared to help you with concerns regarding your child.

"Pick a couple of rules that you always have had that don't change regardless of the circumstance. For example, saying 'please' and 'thank you' when requesting something. Stress the importance of following this rule. This will help give your child a sense of control and accomplishment because they know that they can do this task and always will be able to do this task."

—Mother of a child diagnosed with a brain tumor

80. Can our child attend school during treatment? What can be done to continue our child's education if school attendance isn't possible?

Every diagnosis and subsequent treatment regimen involves a different degree of patient participation and possible side effects. Upon initial diagnosis, most children are too ill and/or too overwhelmed by the treatment to be emotionally or physically involved in school. You and/or a hospital/clinic staff member should inform the school of your child's diagnosis and make them aware of his or her extended absence. Most schools are extremely helpful in providing the missing work. In some treatment protocols, your child may be able to return to their classes fairly quickly after initial treatment. Each child will react differently to treatment, so it is important to check with your doctor for the initial go-ahead, and also to talk with your child for his or her thoughts about returning to school.

If your child is not emotionally ready or it's not medically appropriate to return to school shortly after diagnosis, a referral for home instruction is initiated by a staff member. Inquire with your oncologist as to who does it at your treatment facility. The amount of time provided by the home instruction teacher will differ depending on your state and district. The time that most children receive home instruction is significantly less than regular school attendance. Nevertheless, children tend to excel under home instruction because the work is tailored to their needs and they benefit from the individual attention.

It is important to encourage your child to keep in contact with classmates and the school while absent. Socialization during your child's development can be as important as education. Depending on the treatment phase, your child may be able to visit school and participate in activities. Talk to the school's administration and continue to update them on your child's progress.

81. When can our child return to school? How can we help him/her prepare to return?

When your child is medically cleared to return to school, the transition to a "normal" routine can be difficult even if your child is feeling well. The side effects of

The transition to a "normal" routine can be difficult.

131

treatment, including hair loss, weight gain or loss, and adjustment to illness may impact your child's desire to return to school. Encourage your child to talk about her/his concerns and fears. Accommodations may be made to help in the transition, such as wearing a hat to school. Some clinics/hospitals have a school re-entry program that can help facilitate a smooth transition for your child. This may involve a member of the hospital/clinic staff educating school administration, staff, or classmates about your child's illness. The school re-entry facilitator should work with you and your child to determine what information is to be shared and with whom. Take steps to prepare your child to answer questions about the illness in language that he or she are comfortable using. Role-play potential questions and encourage your child to be as honest as possible with the other students. Depending on your child's comfort level, you may suggest that he or she incorporates the experience or aspects of treatment within the school curriculum (e.g., show and tell, science project, etc.).

Regardless of your current financial situation and your child's age at diagnosis, financial assistance and college scholarships may be available to your child as a result of his or her diagnosis. Scholarships vary by size, criteria, and purpose. A listing of national scholarships is available in the Appendix. Please speak to your clinic's social worker to inquire about additional financial assistance.

82. How can we help make hospital stays easier for our child?

Many treatment protocols will involve hospital stays. Often, infections, bleeds, or fevers will subject your child to an inpatient admission. The hospital can be a scary place for children and adults. The unfamiliar sights, sounds, and environment may evoke feelings of fear and dread. In addition, patients have indicated a dislike of the food, the difficulties in finding quiet, and feelings of loneliness and isolation. However, there are steps that parents can take to help insure that your child's hospital stay is as pleasant as possible. Although not all children find hospitalization to be unpleasant, the provided tips can always augment the experience.

Linens from home can often help personalize the hospital bed and create a less emotionally sterile environment. Hanging pictures and decorating the walls can help make the surroundings more pleasant. Whenever possible, arrange to stay the night with your child. Most pediatric floors will help accommodate your family's wishes to be close to your child and will allow you to stay overnight. If possible, bring food from home or order in from a restaurant. Most children, especially those on chemotherapy, can become easily nauseated by the sights and sounds of unfamiliar food, that is, hospital cafeteria food. Encourage your child to have friends and family visit regularly to help pass the time. Teenagers can often be given permission to wear their street clothes, rather than hospital gowns or pajamas, which may help them feel more comfortable.

"We decided by day 2 of admission to the hospital that we needed to make his room look as familiar and comfortable as possible. We brought 'home' to the hospital. We spread a cozy blanket on his bed, set up books on the windowsill, displayed his toys within reach, and few favorite stuffed animals lived on his bed. We listened to music to create a kid-friendly atmosphere and to drown out the noises of an active hospital. Also, my husband and I were able to spend the night in the hospital. That continuity was paramount

in our experience to reassure our son that he was well loved and would not be abandoned in his time of need."

—Parent of a child diagnosed with ALL

"Contacting organizations, like Children's Brain Tumor Foundation, can help put you in contact with other people in similar situations who can share things that did and didn't work."

—Mother of a child diagnosed with a brain tumor

83. What can we do if eating habits change?

There are many strategies that parents might try to improve oral intake during therapy. However, issues surrounding eating may be a source of conflict during this critical time. A gentle approach and knowing when to apply these strategies are critical. For example, it is impractical to expect children to eat when receiving high-dose chemotherapy. However, when blood counts recover, usually during the week preceding the next course of chemotherapy, children will feel better and be more motivated to eat nutritious foods with a high caloric content. It is also a good idea *not* to offer favorite foods while chemotherapy is being given since some children will develop food aversions.

Be creative with food choices and flexible on eating times.

Be creative with food choices and flexible on eating times. Most children experience weight gain and voracious appetites when taking steroids, which may accompany some treatment protocols. It may be advantageous to offer small frequent snacks and to encourage high-calorie, protein-packed beverages between regular meals (e.g., Boost, Ensure, or Pediasure). Some children may lose interest in favorite foods, so experiment with new foods. When children are nauseated, it may be problematic to insist on regular meals or even snacks. In this case, offer clear liquids at room temperature that may be taken in small sips. It is best to avoid foods with strong odors. Try solid foods three to four hours before any treatment that is associated with nausea. If mouth sores occur, your child's eating will most likely be affected. A major focus will then be on ensuring adequate hydration, but if possible, soft bland foods seem to be best tolerated when mouth sores are present. A nutritionist may be contacted to assist with meal planning if concerns or questions arise.

If serious weight loss develops despite the suggested measures, your physician might consider **nasogastric or gastrostomy feeding**. In these cases, a small tube is placed through the nose into the stomach or intestinal tract ("NG" or "NJ" feeding), or through a tube inserted directly into the stomach through a small incision into the skin (gastrostomy or "G-tube"). It must be recognized that these are temporary measures to ensure nutritional balance. If all these measures fail, intravenous feeding called **total parenteral nutrition** might be necessary.

Nasogastric or gastrostomy feeding

a temporary measure in which a patient is fed through a small tube placed in the stomach or intestines to increase caloric intake.

Total parenteral nutrition

intravenous feeding.

84. How do we help our child cope with hair loss resulting from chemotherapy?

A child's reaction to hair loss tends to be unique to the individual. Adolescents and/or girls tend to have the most difficulty dealing with the loss of hair. It is helpful to introduce the concept of hair loss early in the treatment process. Preparing your child for the inevitable loss will help him or her devise a plan to deal with it. Encourage the child to take "control" by cutting his or her own hair before it falls out.

Children can use the opportunity to try a haircut that they have always wanted. Some children draw on their heads or encourage family or friends to decorate their bald heads after the hair loss. Hats and scarves can be used as well. Other children opt for a wig or partial hair piece. There are many alternative hair pieces available, including hair that is appropriate and comfortable for younger children. There are pediatric cancer programs that provide wigs or hair pieces free of charge. Some insurance policies cover the costs. For the best chance of coverage, ask your child's oncologist to write a prescription for a hair prosthesis. Many children, especially younger children, opt to wear a cap or nothing at all.

Your child may be forced to confront ridicule or stares due to his or her hair loss and/or appearance changes. Although this is often uncomfortable and embarrassing, it can be helpful to use this as an opportunity to talk about accepting others who might be different. As stated earlier, cancer is a disease of physical and emotional consequences. Being prepared for this reality does not make it disappear but it may make it easier to cope with when it arises.

85. Should our child be in private therapy as a result of the diagnosis?

As indicated earlier, a cancer diagnosis is an obvious stressor in the lives of all those affected. The degree and extent to which a patient integrates and adapts to the diagnosis is influenced by many variables. Although the support and care from you as well as concerned family and friends is helpful, there are many times when professional interventions are beneficial for your child. Providing your child with the opportunity to voice his or her concerns, fears, and feelings with a neutral, experienced professional may be advisable.

In many instances, the adjustment to illness period and acute episodes of stress and crisis can be managed by ancillary services, such as behavioral therapists, working with your oncologist. However, there are instances where your child may require more intense or more frequent support services than your treatment center can offer. In addition, your child may have difficulty feeling safe discussing concerns and fears with individuals at the center where they are actively undergoing treatment. In these instances, it may be helpful to access a therapist in your community. Discuss your thoughts with the behavioral health members on staff at your clinic and ask them to help direct you.

"We decided that our child would benefit from the support of a therapist knowledgeable about oncology. The unexpected benefit was to us as parents. The therapist guides and supports us too. She answers every single one of our questions, anxieties, and concerns with compassion and insight, which helps us to navigate the difficult journey."

—Mother of a young child diagnosed with leukemia

86. How will diagnosis and treatment affect our teenager?

It is always important to understand that each individual is different. However, there is extensive literature that identifies the general ways in which children, teenagers in particular, are affected by a diagnosis of cancer and its consequential interruption in "normal" development.

There are many development stages and subsequent maturational tasks that are negotiated on the road to adulthood. Adolescence is a period of time, identified as ages 12 to 19, in which specific areas of independence and individual identity are developed. Issues related to self-esteem, development of a personal value system, acceptance of body image, integration of sexual identity, career plans, and separation and individuation are all addressed during this period.

Adolescents with cancer often experience some loss of self-esteem because they are thrust into an unfamiliar role during a period of time when familiarity has been demonstrated to be of importance. A diagnosis can contribute to a perception of being different that may lead to feelings of inferiority as well. Many of the prescribed treatments and the diagnosis itself affect body image, specifically hair loss, weight gain due to steroid use, and weight loss. Changes in body image, disruption in normal activities due to the diagnosis, and reactions from prescribed therapies can have severe effects on body image, particularly with teens struggling with their sexuality and their rapidly changing bodies. In addition, permanently altered physical presentation as a result of radiation, concerns over sterility and fertility, the ability to bear children, and impotency are all additional concerns that adolescents must address—issues that usually don't surface until adulthood. In addition, many of the effects of treatment—for example, hair and muscle loss—tend to eliminate a teenager's individual opportunities for self-expression and relegate them to looking similar to other diagnosed teens.

Many teenagers are used to fending for themselves and are struggling to identify themselves as separate entities from their family. An illness renders them much more reliant and dependent on their family. Often, much of their independence is recanted as parents become overly concerned with their teen's physical and mental health, and their social activities are subsequently limited.

87. What can I do to help our teenager cope with his or her diagnosis?

As outlined in Question 86, struggling with the developmental tasks associated with adolescence can be very emotionally trying to a teenager. These tasks become more overwhelming when compounded with a diagnosis of a chronic illness. Therefore, it is important to be sensitive to your teen's rapidly changing emotions and reactions to this critical period in his or her life. Listen to your teen's feelings and attempt to validate them. Attempt to understand the appropriate need for separation and individuation while maintaining the new role of patient—someone who is suddenly reliant on his/her parents when feeling ill and subject to the decisions of a medical team. Individuation is a flexible stage of development when the young person attempts different behaviors to express thoughts and feelings, some of which may be uncomfortable experiences for his/her parents. Whenever possible, attempt to include your teenager in discussions regarding their own medical care. Teens will let you know if they are not interested

Include your teenager in discussions regarding their own medical care.

in the discussions. In addition, allow them to make decisions regarding their care when applicable. Instilling a sense of personal control is helpful for all patients. Try to resist being over-protective or unnecessarily limiting their activities. When medically appropriate, encourage them to socialize with their friends and maintain as "normal" a routine as possible. Empower them by making them responsible for taking their medications, and encourage them to follow their protocol and to be aware of impending treatment. When possible, encourage teens to seek out connections with other patients. It may be possible for your child to join a peer support group and/or connect with others who have undergone a similar experience.

"My wife and I spoke with my 12-year-old son at the time of diagnosis. We let him talk about whatever he wanted to...he chose not to read, hear, or talk about it. My other son was also very supportive. He chose to shave his head in support of his kid brother. We joke about the diagnosis a lot as well. Talk to your child and keep them in positive attitude and spirit."

—Father of an adolescent diagnosed with leukemia

---

88. How do we explain this diagnosis to our (other) children, and how can we help them cope?

Many of the suggestions outlined in Question 77 will hold true for explanations to siblings. It is important to remember to use age-appropriate language when speaking with your children about their sibling's diagnosis. Overwhelming children with information that they are unable to comprehend is confusing and scary. Attempt to engage your children in a discussion around the diagnosis and its impact on their lives. Reassure them that the diagnosis is not their fault and that they had no way to cause or stop it. Depending on your child's age, development, and comprehension, the so-called "magical thinking" may lead them to believe that they had some sort of power or control in their brother or sister's diagnosis. For example, remind them that "wishing your bratty little brother would just go away" will not cause an illness. It is also helpful to let them know that the cancer is not contagious.

Invite your other children to the clinic or treatment center if you believe that it would help them feel more involved. Remind them of how important they are to you and why your attention and time may be shifted to their sick sibling at this time. Highlight their role in the family as you all work together to help their brother or sister get better. If you think that you could use the support or skills of a professional, ask for assistance with delivering the information from your oncologist and his/her staff.

Your attention and time will most likely be shifted or occupied during this critical period. This shift in attention can impact your other children, and they may have strong, yet appropriate, reactions and feelings about this change. For example, siblings could be scared that this will happen to them, and some may wish that it would because then they would have the additional attention now given to the ill child. Some siblings may become angry at losing mommy or daddy's time or that their baseball game was missed.

Realize that children react in their own ways and at their own pace. Your child may be unable or slow to articulate their concerns regarding the diagnosis. Feelings may be expressed indirectly. For example, the siblings' behavior may change, causing them to become more withdrawn or to act out, and they may misbehave to get attention.

Use this time as an opportunity to discuss your child's feelings in general, with an emphasis on listening to what he or she needs to say.

It is helpful to let your children know that they can speak to anyone they feel comfortable with about their concerns. A child may have difficulty expressing his or her fears or thoughts about their brother or sister's diagnosis directly to their parent. A trusted adult such as a teacher, family member, medical professional, and/or clergyperson can also be a resource for your child. Support staff at your child's clinic, such as the Child Life Program staff and social workers, can be utilized as well. Find out if your clinic or hospital offers groups or services targeting the unique needs of siblings.

Do your best to maintain consistency and normalcy.

Do your best to maintain consistency and normalcy. Keeping your child in a consistent environment can help him or her maintain their routine and feel safe. For example, see if you can have people come to your home to watch your children if you will be the hospital for extended stays, rather than making your children relocate. Remind your child that this is a difficult time for everyone and that you will do your best to be as available as possible.

89. How do we cope as a couple?

It is very apparent that a cancer diagnosis can potentially place strain on the family, particularly the relationships within and among family members. The relationship between guardians/parents, if existent, is often strained. The focus is no longer on bonding and sharing time together, but rather on the ill child. Your relationship is not the priority as you attempt to hold yourself and your family together. The limited amounts of energy that you possess are generally reserved in attempts at organizing your home. Most relations between parents suffer as a result. This is a general pattern that has been noted, although there are always exceptions. In some case, parents discover that a stronger bond is forged between them as a result of the experience.

Make the effort to create time and space for your "couplehood." Although it is easier said than done, your child will ultimately benefit from the enhanced connection between her or his caregivers. Finding opportunities to go out for dinner, exercise together, or create special windows of time to be alone as a couple can help to normalize the experience for your child and can help you regain your insight and focus when needed. Use your existing support systems—or create them—to help organize a schedule that will allow you a "break" from the routine, but will ensure you have confidence and security in your child's caregiver. Your support systems can include adult family members, friends, or volunteers from different organizations such as religious or cancer support groups. Most importantly, talk with your partner and allow for individual styles of coping and dealing with the experience. Everyone processes the experience differently, and understanding what your partner needs can minimize feelings of hurt and rejection, which may result in a decreased interest in intimacy.

"Find one nice thing to say to each other each day. Even if it means saying, 'Honey, you changed that bandage nicely.'"

—Mother of a young child diagnosed with leukemia

90. How can I help myself cope through this difficult time?

This will be a stressful time for the whole family. As a parent or caregiver, you will be pulled in many directions and you will likely be overwhelmed by the stress, concern, and responsibilities of care. The best way to be available to your child and family is by taking care of yourself. Make an effort to utilize all of the resources around you. This is a very important time to take advantage of people's generosity and offers for assistance. The emotional and physical toll of caring for an ill child is draining and demanding.

Group and individual therapy, offered through your clinic, hospital, private practitioner, and/or local chapters of cancer support organizations (see Appendix), can provide effective tools and a cathartic release to help combat some of the stressors. Utilizing the expertise of "others who have gone before you" and networking with other parents at the clinic is recommended and can also be an invaluable tool. Take this opportunity to listen to yourself and your own body. Find out what you need to best cope with stressful situations and make every effort to maximize on opportunities to utilize it.

"I cope with this very difficult time by making my son laugh a lot and keeping his spirits as high as I can get them. I cry sometimes when I am alone and it is good for me. We try to keep life as normal as possible when possible."

—Father of an adolescent diagnosed with leukemia

91. Should we tell our family and friends about the diagnosis?

It is very difficult for most parents to initially accept and fully understand their child's diagnosis. Some have immediate conflicting feelings. They struggle between protecting themselves and their child from unwanted inquiries and gossip, and wanting to initiate talking about the diagnosis to avoid such inquiries. Any and all of these emotions and feelings are normal. The manner in which you and your family decide to tell family and friends is an individual decision.

All of these emotions and feelings are normal.

However, this journey is impossible to travel alone. Most treatment protocols are rigorous and timely. You and your child's physical and emotional stamina will be constantly tested. A parent(s) must be available to change plans or reschedule on a moment's notice. It will be necessary to draw on all assistance offered in order to be available to your child's erratic treatment schedule and/or your other children's demanding routines. Once people in your life know about the diagnosis and its implications to your family's lifestyle, they may make themselves more available to help with day-to-day assistance. In addition, your friends and family can help to provide the emotional support necessary to get you through the experience.

It is also helpful to remember that this diagnosis is nothing to be ashamed or embarrassed about. Modeling open communication for children will help them to see the benefits of talking about their experiences, as well as help them to normalize the situation.

"I highly recommend that you tell your family and friends about it. You will need the emotional support as a parent. The love and support that comes from our family and friends is what keeps us sane as well as financially sound. Know from the start of this journey that there is not anything that you did or didn't do that caused this to happen to your loved one."

—Father of a child diagnosed with leukemia

"People have been very understanding. When they ask how my son is doing, I make a sincere attempt to give them an optimistic progress report."

—Mother of a child diagnosed with leukemia

92. Are we protected if we take a leave of absence from work to care for our child?

Family Medical Leave Act (FMLA)

A legislative act that allows eligible employees to take up to 12 work weeks per year of unpaid leave to care for their ill family member (immediate family only). Employees will maintain their group health coverage, and after returning from leave will keep the same job position or an equal position within the employer's company.

The **Family Medical Leave Act (FMLA)** was designed to assist families in balancing the demands of the workplace with the needs of the family. The Act states (according to the U.S. Department of Labor), "covered employers must grant an eligible employee up to a total of 12 work weeks for unpaid leave during any 12-month period for several, specified reasons." The applicable reason, as it pertains to this issue, is to care for an immediate family member (spouse, child, or parent) with a serious health condition. Parents or caregivers may request a leave from their jobs, as long as they have been employed by the employer for at least 12 months, for at least 1,250 hours of service during the 12-month period immediately preceding the leave, and are employed at a worksite where 50 or more employees are employed by the employer within

75 miles of the worksite. Medical records are not required for leave, but medical verification may be required by your employer. The leave does not need to be continuous. Although employees will not be paid for their leave time, they will maintain coverage under their group health plan, and they will be guaranteed restoration to the same or equivalent position when they return to work. When possible or foreseeable, at least 30 days advance notice is requested before leave commences. There should be no applicable penalty under FMLA. A social worker at your treatment facility can help provide you with more information.

"I have found that explaining my son's illness to colleagues at work has created a strong atmosphere of empathy. But I am very conscious about not using my situation at home as an excuse for any reason, when I have difficulty meeting a deadline or I might be absent from work."

—Mother of a young child diagnosed with ALL

---

93. We have heard of cancer support organizations. What are their functions?

Organizations provide education and individual counseling, group counseling, Internet support, and/or telephone support groups. (Some facilities have staff that speak different languages.) Some organizations offer introductions to patients with the same diagnosis, or who have completed a similar experience, who can offer support and insight. Some of the groups offer support to distinct populations based on diagnosis, region of the country, and/or the relationship to the patient (i.e., caregiver, sibling).

The larger organizations, such as Cancer Care, American Cancer Society, Candlelighter's Childhood Cancer Foundation, The Children's Cancer Association, and the National Children's Cancer Society, have many branches throughout the country and world, and offer emotional support to families regardless of specific diagnosis. Most referrals are initiated by social workers, but many organizations welcome inquiries directly from families as well. The Leukemia and Lymphoma Society and the Children's Brain Tumor Foundation cater specifically to providing support to their respective, specific diagnoses. There are many local, smaller organizations that can be helpful as well. For a complete list and contact information, please see the Appendix.

94. Will our insurance cover everything?

Every insurance policy is different, so it is important to understand your policy and its referral procedures. Individual policies work differently when it comes to treatment coverage. Chemotherapies and medications are not always covered under your plans, especially if you have a limited policy. Talk to your social worker about the possibility of applying for additional coverage, which can be available based on financial status or diagnosis. It is important to know which insurances are accepted where your child is undergoing treatment as well as facilities where you are being referred for additional tests, scans, and blood work. Please note that not all facilities affiliated with the hospital or clinic will participate with your insurance plan. You can ask your doctor if there are alternatives or options that are covered within your plan. Most importantly, stay on top of your bills and follow up on all referrals. By catching a potential problem in billing or coverage early, you can possibly avoid future out-of-pocket expenses. If a hospital financial counselor is available, it may be helpful to set up an appointment with him or her to determine your specific coverage situation.

95. Are there financial resources available to us and our child?

There are many organizations available that provide financial, counseling, and information/referral assistance to the families of children with cancer (see Appendix). Levels of assistance are often based on the area of the country in which you live, personal financial resources, and type of cancer. Many of the organizations offer one-time grants, while others are available for assistance as needs arise. The grants usually assist with unanticipated costs or those not covered by insurance. These may include transportation and parking for the hospital, co-payments on medication, and/or food for inpatient stays. Some organizations require financial information, including bank statements, to apply. Ask your social worker for availability of assistance in your area (see Appendix).

Children, with their parents' assistance, can also apply for Social Security disability benefits as a result of their diagnosis. These benefits are available based on financial status and level of disability. Call 1-800-772-1213 in the United States to determine whether your child is a candidate to receive these benefits.

"There are wonderful agencies out there that are more than happy to help you. The Leukemia and Lymphoma Society, Cancer Care, Friends of Karen, and others. The social workers are also very helpful and will answer any questions and even dig deeper then your question to assist you. Be certain to utilize any assistance available to you and don't let pride stand in your way. It helps to have help."

—Father of an adolescent diagnosed with leukemia

96. What if we live far from the treating facility?

When families live far from treating facilities, alternative, temporary living arrangements can sometimes be made. Ronald McDonald houses, which offer temporary living arrangements at minimal costs for the family and patient, are located in many cities throughout the country. Additionally, more localized options for accommodations may be available. Certain hospitals and clinics have arrangements with local hotels that offer discount rates for short stays. In some cases, charitable organizations can absorb the cost of temporary housing. Talk with your social worker and explore the options available in your city.

97. Can our child have a pet during treatment?

During treatment, your child's immune system may become compromised. This compromised immune system may result in greater susceptibility to infection. This susceptibility will be most prevalent during the initial phase of treatment and when your child's white blood cell count has dropped due to treatment (see Question 51 about neutropenia). Although most organisms and germs carried by household pets are not harmful to humans, the chances of infection increase when your child is ill or on treatment. You should avoid more exotic pets like turtles, reptiles, and parrots, as they may carry particularly troublesome infections.

The chances of infection increase when your child is ill or on treatment.

Doctors' opinions may differ slightly, but most would not recommend that children give up their cat or dog during this extremely emotional and fragile period in their lives. In fact, "pet therapy" is being integrated into the treatment of many chronic diseases, including cancer, because of the emotional wellness associated with animal contact. However, your child may need to limit contact with the animal and avoid daily maintenance and care of the animal. They should not change the litter box or clean up after the pet. The animal should be well groomed and be up to date on all vaccinations. Children should avoid any roughhousing or playing that would encourage scratches or bites from the pet. For that reason, the optimal time for introducing a new puppy or kitten is after periods of neutropenia have resolved. If your oncologist supports your child's interaction with his or her pet, you should encourage the comforting relationship.

98. Are summer vacation opportunities available to our child?

A pediatric diagnosis of cancer, or any other life-threatening disease, is an intrusion on the lives of all those affected. Many of their chances for a "normal" childhood, filled with opportunities for bonding with their peers, socializing, and "care free" fun are greatly limited. However, programs exist that have been designed in consideration of the specific needs of your child.

Summer camp programs, which cater specifically to children with cancer and chronic illness, provide a unique opportunity for children to interact with other children with similar diagnoses. Camps catering to children with chronic illness offer qualified, on-site medical staff familiar with various diagnoses and related treatment. The activities and camp structure are designed with the child's needs and limitations in mind. Almost all of these camps are free of charge to families who attend. Each camp is different in design and length of the program, and the organization varies. Additionally, certain camps are available for family members of the diagnosed child as well as the patient themselves. A listing of camps can be found in the Appendix. Please speak with your social worker and oncologist about suitable camps available to your child and family.

99. When should our child resume "normal activities" after treatment has begun?

Once your child begins treatment, he/she may experience periods where the body's immunity is extremely low. During these periods, it is advisable to avoid crowds, excessive exposure to public places, and areas of high traffic with many people. Your doctor can determine these times through a routine blood test. However, when your child is not immune-suppressed, maintaining a schedule similar to one before diagnosis can be extremely beneficial.

A diagnosis of cancer greatly affects a child, family, and their daily routine. Any attempts or effort at maintaining a normalized routine is comforting for the child. Minimizing the effect of the diagnosis and its interference with everyone's daily life can help everyone adjust more quickly to the overall program. Whenever possible, attempt to include the faces and places that were familiar in your child's life prior to diagnosis. Facilitate interaction between your child, friends, schoolmates, and family.

100. Where can we find more information about pediatric cancer?

Additional information and resources on pediatric cancers can be found in the Appendix of this book. Your pediatric oncology team will have contacts with local resources and will be aware of special events, education opportunities, and ongoing support groups held in your region. Networking among other families who have a family member undergoing cancer treatment, in remission, or has been cancer-free for a number of years may prove to be invaluable resources. The Appendix lists some Web sites that have been reviewed and have been considered helpful to other families. Be aware that some Internet Web sites promote anecdotal or incorrect information. Always review internet findings or stories with your medical team. As always, when you have a question about your child's care, it is important to communicate with your pediatric oncologist and his or her medical team.

The authors of this book do not endorse any organizations listed, nor guarantee that individuals will qualify for the services that they provide. Please contact each organization for their specific criteria. This is not a complete list of all resources. Speak to your social worker or oncologist's team to determine whether there are local organizations that may be available to provide support or assistance.

General Financial Assistance/ Support Organizations

American Brain Tumor Foundation
2720 River Road, Ste 146
Des Plaines, IL 60018
Voice: 800-886-2282 or 847-827-9910
Fax: 847-827-9918
www.abta.org

American Cancer Society (ACS)
1599 Clifton Rd., NE
Atlanta, GA 30329
Voice: 800-ACS-2345
Fax: 404-325-2217
www.cancer.org

Cancer Care, Inc.
275 7th Avenue
New York, NY 10001
Voice: 800-813-HOPE
Fax: 212-719-0263
www.cancercare.org

Cancer Fund of America

Eastern Region
2901 Breezewood Lane
Knoxville, TN 37921-1099
Voice: 865-938-5284
Fax: 865-938-2968
www.cfoa.org

Western Region
2223 N. 56th Street
Knoxville, NY 37921
Voice: 408-654-4715

Candlelighter's Childhood Cancer Foundation
3910 Warren Avenue
P.O. Box 498
Kensington, MD 20895-0498
Voice: 800-366-2223 or 301-962-3520
Fax: 301-962-3521
www.candlelighters.org

Catholic Charities, USA
1731 King St.
Alexandria, VA 22314
Voice: 703-549-1390
Fax: 703-549-1656
www.catholiccharitiesusa.org

Chai Lifeline
Health support services for seriously ill Jewish children and their
    families.
151 West 30th Street
New York, NY 10001
Voice: 212-465-1300
Fax: 212-465-0949
www.chailifeline.org

Children's Brain Tumor Foundation
274 Madison Avenue, Suite 130
New York, NY 10016
Voice: 212-448-9494
Fax: 212-448-1022
www.cbtf.org

Cure for Lymphoma Foundation
1731 King St.
Alexandria, VA 22314
Voice: 800-CFL-6848 or 212-213-9595
Fax: 703-549-1656

First Hand Foundation
c/o Cermer Corp.
2800 Rockcreek Parkway
Kansas City, MO 64117
Voice/Fax: 816-201-1569
www.firsthandfoundation.org

Friends of Karen
P.O. Box 190
118 Titicus Rd.
Purdys, NY 10578
914-277-4547
Fax: 914-277-4967

Hill-Burton Funds
Federal assistance is available to those who are unable to pay, and
is provided by the Hill-Burton Act of Congress. Public and
nonprofit hospitals, nursing homes, and other medical facilities
may provide subsidized low-cost or no-cost medical care to ful-
fill their community service obligation.
Voice: 800-638-0742
TDD: 800-537-7697
http://www.hhs.gov/ocr

Hip Hat
Hats with hair and wig alternative head gear.
108 W. Adalee Street
Tampa, Florida
Voice: 877-447-4287
www.hip-hat.com

The Lance Armstrong Foundation
P.O. Box 161150
Austin, TX 78716
(512) 236-8820
www.laf.org

The Leukemia and Lymphoma Society
600 Third Avenue
New York, NY 10016
800-995-4LSA
Fax: 212-856-9686
www.leukemia.org

Locks of Love
Provides hairpieces to financially challenged children suffering
    from long-term (permanent) medical hair loss.
1640 S. Congress Avenue, Suite 104
Palm Springs, FL 33461
561-963-1677 and 888-896-1588
Fax: 561-963-9914
www.locksoflove.org

National Children's Cancer Society (NCCS)
1015 Locust, Suite 600
St. Louis, MO 63101
800-532-6459
Fax: 314-241-6949
www.children-cancer.com

Pharmaceutical Manufacturers' Association
Patient assistance programs for those who cannot afford
    prescriptions
1100 Fifteenth St. NW
Washington, D.C. 20005
Voice: 800-762-4636
www.helpingpatients.org

Ronald McDonald House Charities
Temporary housing for families of seriously ill children being
    treated away from home.
1 Knock Drive, Dept. 014
Oak Brook, IL 60521
630-623-7048
www.rmhc.org

Sick Kids Need Involved People

Information and assistance to families of children with complex
   medical needs.
213 W. 35th Street, Floor 11
New York, NY 10001
212-268-5999
Fax: 212-268-7667

Social Security Administration (SSA)

Office of Public Inquiries
Windsor Park Building
6401 Security Blvd.
Baltimore, MD 21235
Voice: 800-772-1213
www.ssa.gov

Clinical Trials / General Cancer Information

CancerNet

http://cancernet.nci.nih.gov
This site provides accurate cancer information, including the
   Physicians Data Query (PDQ), which is the National Cancer
   Institute's comprehensive cancer database.

Children's Oncology Group Web Site

www.childrensoncologygroup.org
This site provides general information about childhood cancer as
   well as treatment protocols.

National Cancer Institute

Cancer Information Source
1–800–4–CANCER
1–800–332–8615 (for the hearing impaired)

CancerTrials web site: http://cancertrials.nci.nih.gov
This site provides comprehensive clinical trials information.

Medical Air Travel

American Airlines—Miles for Kids
PO Box 619616, Mail Drop 2705
Fort Worth, TX 76155
Voice: 817-963-8118 ext. 4
Fax: 817-931-6890

Angel Flight America
National Headquarters
P.O. Box 17467
Memphis, TN 38187
For requests: 800-446-1231
For donation: 877-621-7177
Flights less than 1000 miles

Corporate Angel Network Program
Westchester County Airport
1 Loop Road, Building 1
White Plains, NY 10604
Voice: 914-328-1313
www.corporateangelnetwork.org

Delta SkyWish/United Way of America
701 N. Fairfax Street
Alexandria, VA 22314-2045
Voice: 703-836-7112
800-892-2757 ext.285
www.valleyunitedway.org/skywich.html

Mercy Medical Airlift
4620 Haygood Road, Suite 1
Virginia Beach, VA 23455
Voice: 757-318-9174
Flights more than 1,000 miles

National Patient Air Transport Helpline
PO Box 1940
Manassas, VA 20108-0804
www.npath.org

Wish Granting Organizations

Wish fulfillment organizations grant a variety of wishes to children with a chronic or life-threatening illness. Eligibility requirements differ among organizations.

Children's Wish Foundation International
P.O. Box 28785
Atlanta, GA 30350-1822
Voice: 1-800-323-WISH
www.childrenswish.org

Make-A-Wish Foundation of America
3550 North Central Ave.
Suite 300
Phoenix, AZ 85012-2127
Voice: 800-722-9474
Fax: 602-279-9474
www.wish.org

Marty Lyons Foundation, Inc.
326 West 48th Street
New York, NY 10036
Voice: 212-977-9474
www.martylyonsfoundation.org

Starlight Children's Foundation
5900 Wilshire Blvd., Suite 2530
Los Angeles, CA 90036
Voice: 310-207-5558 or 800-247-7827
Fax: 323-634-0090
www.starlight.org

Scholarship Resources Information

Access Foundation
Foundation for the Disabled
www.anova.org/access

American Cancer Society
1599 Clifton Rd., NE
Atlanta, GA 30329
Voice: 800-ACS-2345
Atlanta office: 404-320-3333
Texas office: 512-919-1886
Fax: 404-325-2217
www.cancer.org

Cancer Survivors' Scholarship Fund
P.O. Box 792
Missouri City, TX 77459
Voice: 281-437-9505
Fax: 281-437-9568
www.cancersurvivorsfund.org

Federal Student Aid Information Center
P.O. Box 84
Washington, D.C. 20044-0084
Voice: 800-4-FED-AID or 1-800-433-3243
www.fafsa.ed.gov

Health Resources Center
1 Dupont Circle
Washington, DC 20036
1-800-544-3284
www.advocacycenter.org

Matt Stauffer Memorial Scholarship
One $1000 yearly scholarship awarded
PMB #505
4725 Dorsey Hall Dr. Suite A
Ellicott City, MD 21402
1-888-393-FUND or 410-964-0202
www.ulmanfund.org

National Amputation Foundation
One $250 scholarship
12-45 150th Street
Whitestone, NY 11357
Voice: 718-767-0596
www.nationalamputation.org

Novartis Scholarships for Students with Immune Deficiencies
Voice: 800-926-4433
www.Novartis.com

Scholarship 58
Eight $5000 yearly scholarships awarded
Patient Advocate Foundation
753 Thimble Shoals Blvd., Suite B
Newport News, VA 23606
www.collegescholarships.com

Camps for Children Diagnosed with Cancer

Camp Mak-A-Dream
Children's Oncology Camp Foundation
P.O. Box 1450
Missoula, MT 59806
Voice: 406-549-0987
www.campdream.org

Camp Simcha
National Headquarters
151 30th Street
New York, NY 10001
Voice: 877-CHAI-LIFE/212-465-0949
www.chailifeline.org/camp_simcha.asp

Camp Sunshine
35 Acadia Road
Casco, ME 04015
Voice: 207-655-3800
www.campsunshine.org

Hole in the Wall Gang Camp
565 Ashford Center Road
Ashford, CT 06278
Voice: 860-429-7295
www.holeinthewallgang.org

Appendix

The Silver Lining Foundation
1490 Ute Avenue
Aspen, CO 81611
Voice: 970-925-9540
www.silverliningfoundation.org

Special Love, Inc. (Camp Fantastic)
117 Youth Development Court
Winchester, VA 22602
Voice: 540-667-3774
www.speciallove.org

Glossary

Absolute neutrophil count (ANC): Determined through routine blood draw to estimate risk of infection. Neutrophils are white blood cells that are formed in bone marrow tissue and protect against infection.

Acute lymphomblastic leukemia (ALL): A form of cancer that starts in the white blood cells; poorly developed cells (called blast cells) grow and multiply in an uncontrolled way in the bone marrow; they replace normal bone marrow cells and spread throughout the body. Symptoms can include severe anemia, hemorrhages, and a slight enlargement of the lymph nodes, liver, or spleen.

Acute myelocytic leukemia (AML): A type of cancer that starts with a defect in the immature cells of bone marrow; myeloblast cells (immature white blood cells) replace red blood cells and the circulating blood spreads the disease. At the same time, the bone marrow cannot make enough normal red blood cells, white blood cells and platelets.

Symptoms include anemia, inability to fight infection, and easy bleeding.

Acute promyelocytic leukemia (APML): A subtype of the acute myelocytic leukemia cancer; abnormal, heavily granulated promyelocytes (a form of white blood cells) accumulate in bone marrow and blood, and replace normal blood cells.

Allogenic: Term used in transplantation that means genetically dissimiliar. Healthy tissue from a parent, sibling, or non-relative will be matched before being transplanted into a patient.

Allotransplant: Tissue or an organ taken from one individual and implanted into another unrelated person.

Anemia: Not enough red blood cells in the blood, which results in insufficient oxygen to the tissues or organs. Symptoms can include fatigue, pale skin, shortness of breath, and heart problems.

Angiogenesis: Development of new blood vessels.

Autologous: Term used in transplantation that means that a patient's own healthy cells are used to stimulate the growth of more healthy cells.

B-cell: A major type of lymphocyte (white blood cell) that helps protect the body from infection.

Benign tumors: Type of solid mass or growth that remains in one spot in the body, does not invade surrounding areas or travel to other areas (metastasize).

Biopsy: A surgical procedure that involves obtaining a tissue specimen from the body for laboratory testing to determine a more precise diagnosis.

Blasts: Immature blood cells or precursor cells.

Blood: The "circulating tissue" of the body; the fluid and its suspended elements that circulates through the heart, arteries capillaries, and veins; the means by which oxygen and nutritive materials are transported to the tissues, and carbon dioxide and toxins are removed for excretion. Blood consists of plasma, where red blood cells, white blood cells, and platelets are suspended.

Bone: The hard connective tissue that forms the skeleton.

Bone marrow: Spongy, internal space of bones where new blood cells are produced on a daily basis.

Bone marrow aspirate: Removal of small volumes of bone marrow. These cells, when examined under microscope, identify any abnormality in developing blood cells.

Bone marrow biopsy: Procedure involving a needle inserted into the bone to remove a solid core of bone marrow.

Bone marrow donor: Person who donates healthy bone marrow. This tissue will be transplanted or transfused into a patient with damaged or diseased bone marrow cells to replace that patient's bone marrow cells and lead to the production of healthy bone marrow.

Bone marrow transplant: Procedure in which a section of bone marrow is taken from one person and transfused into another; used to replace bone marrow that has been damaged or diseased.

Broviac: A type of long-term central venous catheter; a specific type of tubing that is placed through the chest wall into a large blood vessel; used to allow the passage of fluid to flow in or out of the body.

Cancer: General term used to characterize malignant tumors or neoplasms; these cells multiply rapidly and invade surrounding tissues. If untreated, they can metastasize to several sites in the body and cause death in the patient.

Cancer statistics: Ongoing nationwide collection of data about types of cancer, treatment methods, prognosis, and patient outcome that are analyzed and used to develop guidelines for treatment.

Carcinogen: Toxic material or organism in the environment that produces cancer.

Catheter: A tubular instrument inserted into the body to allow the passage of fluids in or out of a body cavity or blood vessel.

Catecholamines: Major biochemical agents involved with the physical response to stress; includes epinephrine, norepinephrine, and L-dopa. Levels are often elevated in neuroblastoma.

Child Life Program: Specialists in childhood development assist the sick child to cope with visits with the doctor in the hospital and different medical procedures. Often play therapy involves toys, magic tricks, art, music, and storytelling.

Chromosome: One of the bodies (normally 46 in humans) in the cell nucleus that is the bearer of genes; is shaped in a delicate filament.

Circadian rhythm: Biological variations with a cycle of about 24 hours.

Cognition: Generic term to describe the mental activities associated with thinking, learning, and memory; any process whereby one acquires knowledge.

Complete blood count (CBC): Test performed on a blood sample that determines the number of red cells,

white cells, and platelets as well as erythrocyte indices and hematocrit.

Cord blood: Blood in a newborn's umbilical chord; it is rich in stem cells and may be stored in a blood bank.

Central nervous system (CNS): pertaining to the brain, cranial nerves, and spinal cord. Nerves are a chord-like structure that bundles in filaments branching throughout the body; carries electrical impulses to signal or stimulate each cell to do its specific task.

Central venous catheters: Small, flexible tube inserted into large vein above the heart through which drugs and blood products can be given and blood samples can be withdrawn virtually painlessly.

Chemotherapy: Drug treatment utilizing chemicals that have a toxic effect on cancer; some are designed to limit cell growth while other types kill specific cells.

Clinical trial: A research study that carefully examines and analyzes the course of a disease in a defined set of human subjects, which has a specific clinical event as an outcome measure. Clinical trials are designed to learn scientifically valid information about the safety and effectiveness of a drug (alone or in combination), diagnostic test, surgical procedure, or other type of medical intervention in the hopes of improving medical care.

Computed tomography (CT): utilizes an x-ray source called tomography that rotates 360° around the patient to produce an image used for clinical diagnostics. Many soft tissue structures not shown by conventional radiography can be seen with CT.

Conscious sedation: A brief deep sleep caused by intravenous medication; often used to avoid pain from a medical procedure.

Cure: Patient having no evidence of disease for a period of time; for some types of cancer this is 5 to 10 years of being cancer-free.

Cytomegalovirus (CMV): A common group of viruses in the Herpesviridae family that affects humans and animals; the virus is usually associated with a mild infection, although it can lead to severe illness in bone marrow transplant patients.

Deoxyribonucleic acid (DNA): Found primarily in the nuclei of animal and plant cells, this type of nucleic acid is involved with the reproduction of the chromosome, and is where hereditary information is stored.

Donor directed product: A blood donation intended for a specific person.

Echocardiogram: A test using high-frequency sound waves to picture the heart and surrounding tissues for diagnostic purposes.

Emla or Elamax crème: A topical anesthetic applied to the skin and used to numb area before a needle is to be inserted.

Family Medical Leave Act (FMLA): A legislative act that allows eligible employees to take up to 12 work weeks per year of unpaid leave to care for their ill family member (immediate family only). Employees will maintain their group health coverage, and after returning from leave will keep the same job position or an equal position within the employer's company.

Food and Drug Administration (FDA): Federal agency that protects public health by regulating the safety and efficacy of food, medical products, biotechnology, and cosmetics. No drug or device can be sold on the market unless it has undergone rigorous scientific testing and passed the strict regulations of the FDA.

Fellow: Graduate from medical school who has completed specialty training in medicine and is completing advanced training in a subspecialty.

Fever: A complex physiologic response to infection or disease, characterized by a rise in core body temperature above normal, usually more than 38°C (100.4°F).

Fraction: Radiology delivered in small increments to avoid damaging cells outside of the tumor or mass.

Gamma knife: A noninvasive surgery using gamma radiation that precisely targets a lesion; most often used for brain tumors and vascular malformations.

Gene: Functional unit of heredity on a specific place (locus) on the chromosome; capable of reproducing itself exactly at each cell division; directs the formation of an enzyme or other protein.

Gene mutation: A defect that occurs within the genetic material and is reproduced in subsequent cell divisions instead of the normal genetic material.

Glucose: The chief source of energy for body tissues; controlled by insulin.

Graft rejection: A situation in which the donated marrow is recognized as foreign and destroyed by the immune system.

Graft vs. host disease: A common and serious complication of bone marrow transplantation where there is a reaction against a patient's own tissue by the donated bone marrow.

Guided imagery: Psychological visualization and breath technique used to help a person relax physically and mentally; often used to counteract symptoms associated with pain and anxiety.

Harvest: Collecting cells, tissues, or organisms.

Hematocrit (Hct): Percentage of the volume of a blood sample that is occupied by red blood cells.

Hemoglobin (Hb): The red respiratory protein of red blood cells (erythrocytes) that transports oxygen from the lungs to the tissues.

Hepatoblastoma/hepatocellular carcinoma: A malignant tumor occurring in the liver.

Human lymphocyte antigen (HLA): Proteins present on cells, important in

immunity, are used to determine the potential success for a matching donor transplantation (such as bone marrow).

Hodgkin disease: Malignant disease of lymph tissues; originates in lymph node and tends to spread to spleen, liver, and/or bone marrow.

Home schooling: Tutoring performed outside of a public or private school for a child who is unable attend due to a specified documented excuse; often takes less time for the child to learn the curriculum because of the individualized attention.

Hospice: An organization that provides physical, psychological, social, and spiritual care for dying persons and their families (see Palliative care).

Hyperdiploidy: A condition in which a person is born with more than 46 chromosomes.

Individuation: Stage of childhood development when the personality is differentiated, developed, and expressed.

Infection: invasion and multiplication of germs in body tissues that potentially cause disease; may be due to germs not commonly observed in healthy individuals.

Inherited mutation: A defect in the gene that is transmitted from parent to child (see Mutation, Gene).

Intensity modulated radiation therapy (IMRT): High precision radiotherapy using computer-controlled x-ray acceleration to deliver precise doses of radiation to a tumor or specific areas within the tumor; used in conjunction with computed tomography.

Intern: Graduate of medical school in the first year of training in a medical specialty.

Intravenous: Within a vein or veins.

Intravenous contrast: Liquid that enhances the differences between two or more cell densities in the body; highlights blood vessels and allows optimal radiological images.

In vitro fertilization: A process whereby (usually multiple) ova are placed in a medium and sperm are added; the resulting zygote is inserted into the uterus and allowed to develop to term.

Leukemia: Progressive multiplication of abnormal leukocytes found in the blood and other organs. Acute symptoms include anemia, hemorrhages, and enlargement of lymph nodes, and/or spleen.

Leukocyte: Type of cell formed in the lymphatic system, bone marrow, and reticuloendothelial system and distributed via the blood; are white blood cells and function to fight infection.

Locus: The specific place on a pair of chromosomes where genes are located.

Lymph nodes: Small round, oval, or bean-shaped bodies located along the length of the lymphatic vessels, a system that produces and stores cells that fight infection.

Lymphomas: Malignant cell growth (neoplasms) in the lymphatic system.

Magnetic resonance imaging (MRI): A radiologic technique that scans the body with radio frequency pulses to generate a three-dimensional picture that is useful for clinical diagnostics.

Malignant: Neoplasms (cancer cells) that are locally invasive and destructive; grow rapidly and metastasize.

Mass: A lump or group of cellular material.

Matched unrelated donor (MUD) transplant: when donor marrow comes from a person outside of the immediate family and is matched using HLA matching.

Medical play: Therapeutic technique used to help children understand their diagnosis and the medical environment. Young children are able to touch and play with certain medical instruments and toys, and/or visit different areas of the hospital under the guidance of a social worker or pediatric specialist, to familiarize them before a procedure.

Medi-port: A type of central venous catheter; device that utilizes a line leading to a reservoir that is located underneath the skin; a needle is inserted into the reservoir to deliver medication (see Catheter)

Metastasis: The spread of cancer to distant spots in the body; for example, the appearance of neoplasms in parts of the body remote from the primary tumor. The cells may be spread by the lymphatic system or blood vessels.

Molecular medicine: The art and science of preventing or curing disease on a molecular level; includes genetic manipulation.

Monoclonal antibodies: Artificially produced anitbodies that recognize specific proteins, allowing them to be aimed only at cancer cells.

Mucositis: Inflammation of a mucous membrane, which is a thin sheet or layer of pliable tissue that lines or envelopes a cavity like the oral cavity.

Mutation: A change in the chemistry of a gene, in the base pairs of the chromosome molecule, which is perpetuated in subsequent divisions of a cell in which it occurs.

Nasogastric or gastronomy feeding: Nutrients are given to a patient through a small tube placed in the stomach or intestines; temporary measure designed to increase caloric intake.

Neoplasm: An abnormal tissue that grows by cellular proliferation more rapidly than normal and continues to grow after the stimuli that caused that new growth ceases.

Neupogen: Medication administered under the skin to assist in increasing the neutrophil count (see Neutrophil).

Neuroblastoma: A malignant neoplasm (cancer) characterized by immature, slightly differentiated nerve cells; occurs frequently in infants and children in the septum areas between two parts of an organ or cavity; can be associated with the adrenal gland and retroperitoneal tissue (located next to the abdominal cavity); widespread metastases to the liver, lungs, lymph nodes, cranial cavity, and skeleton are common.

Neutropenia: Presence of abnormally small numbers of neutrophils (white blood cells) in the circulating blood, increasing the risk of infection; usually is temporary.

Neutrophils: A type of white blood cell found in bone marrow tissue and blood that is a major defense against bacteria and fungal organisms.

Non-Hodgkin lymphoma: Malignant disease of the lymph glands that is other than Hodgkin disease; has a nodular or diffuse tumor pattern and tends to be more widespread in the body when diagnosed; more common in children.

Nurse practitioner: A registered nurse (RN) who has graduated from an accredited nursing school, passed a state license examination, and has advanced training in a particular area of health care.

Oncologist: Graduate of a medical school who has been trained and licensed in the art and science of medicine, who is educated and trained specifically in oncology, which deals with the physical, chemical, and biologic properties and features of neoplasms (cancer), including causation, pathogenesis, and treatment.

Osteosarcoma: Type of cancer that occurs on the surface of bone without an involvement of the bone marrow.

Palliative care: Compassionate care including pain management; seeks to address physical, emotional, social, and spiritual pain to achieve best quality of life for patients and their families.

Pediatrician: Graduate of an accredited medical school, passed a state licensing exam to practice medicine, specializing in the study and treatment of children in health and disease during their development from birth through adolescence.

Peripheral line: Semipermanent intravenous access through a vein in an arm and/or hand for injection of medication.

Petechiae: Minute spots on the skin that are not blanched by pressure; signifies hemorrhage.

Platelets: An irregularly shaped disk-like fragment of a cell that is shed from bone marrow into the blood stream, where it functions in blood clotting.

Polymerase chain reaction (PCR): A method of creating copies of specific fragments of DNA; rapidly amplifies a single DNA molecule into many billions of the same molecule.

Positron emission tomography (PET): A type of imaging technique using a metabolic tracer; active tumor tissue can be seen but not its size; can assess whether masses are made up of viable tumor cells or scar tissues.

Procedural accompaniment: Child Life specialist explains a medical procedure to a patient and guides their use of a new technique.

Protocol: A precise and detailed plan for the study of a biological problem or a particular treatment regimen of therapy.

Radiation therapy: The sending forth of light, short radio waves, ultraviolet, or x-rays, or any other rays for treatment. Technique destroys tumor cells by exposing the affected tissue to radiation; usually consists of daily sessions for several weeks.

Randomization: Assignment of an individual to a particular experimental or control group for a clinical study that is done by chance; this eliminates or lessens any potential bias in the scientific study.

Red blood cells (RBC): Cells in blood that transport oxygen; mature cells are called erythrocytes.

Relaxation breathing: Deep, regular breathing technique associated with a quieting of the mind and body; used in yoga and proven effective to reduce physiologic stress.

Remission: Complete disappearance of the signs and symptoms of a disease in response to treatment or spontaneously.

Resident: Graduate of medical school in the second or third year of training in a specialty area.

Rhabdomyosarcoma: A malignant neoplasm (cancer) derived from skeletal muscle.

"Roadmaps": A calendar of treatment based on scientific data to optimize medical care.

Ronald McDonald House: Temporary low-cost housing accommodations for families and patients with chronic illness who are far from home while receiving treatment at a hospital.

Sarcoma: A connective tissue neoplasm (cancer), usually highly malignant, formed in muscles, bones, or other supporting structures of the body.

School re-entry program: Program designed to facilitate a smooth transition to school after an extended absence of the patient due to illness; generally guided by a Child Life specialist who educates school staff and classmates.

Social Security Disability Insurance (SSD): Federal program that provides cash payments and health care coverage when an adult worker or eligible individual is unable to work for at least one year due to physical or mental impairment.

Social worker: Graduate from an accredited school of social work, having passed a state licensing exam to practice psychological counseling and provide other types of aid to individuals and families.

Sperm bank: Place where sperm are collected and frozen in liquid nitrogen for later use in artificial insemination.

Spinal tap/lumbar puncture: Procedure in which a sample of spinal fluid is extracted in order to test for the presence of tumor cells.

Staging: Identifies the extent of involvement by the primary tumor, where the cancer first developed; used to develop a treatment strategy.

Stem cells: A precursor, undifferentiated cell that can divide into daughter cells that differentiate into other cells; stem cells retain the ability to divide and recycle throughout postnatal (immediately after birth) life.

Sterility: An inability to induce conception and produce offspring.

Subcutaneous: The fatty tissue under the skin; injection of fluid such as liquid medicine or nutrition is often performed with a needle into the subcutaneous area.

Supplemental Security Income (SSI): Federal program that provides cash payments and health care coverage when a child (under 18) has a medically determinable impairment(s) that causes marked and severe functional limitations.

T-cells: A major type of lymphocyte (white blood cell) formed in lymph cells that helps protect body from foreign substances; responsible for cell-mediated immunity.

Therapeutic interventions: Treatment of a disease or disorder using clinical and/or psychological methods designed to help the body and/or person heal physically and/or emotionally.

Thrombocytopenia: A condition where there is an abnormally small number of platelets in the circulating blood; may be associated with metastatic neoplasms (cancer), tuberculosis, leukemia, or with suppression of bone marrow.

Total parenteral nutrition: Intravenous feeding.

Transducer: Device that converts one type of energy to another.

Transfusion: Introduction of whole blood or blood component from one individual (donor) directly into another individual (recipient) via the blood stream.

Transplantation: Procedure that transfers tissue or an organ from one part to another in the body, or from one individual (donor) to another (recipient). Also called grafting.

Tumor: An abnormal swelling, growth, or mass (neoplasm) of tissue in the body; may be benign (does not form metastases, and does not invade or destroy adjacent tissue) or malignant (invades surrounding tissues, capable of producing metastases, and may recur after attempted removal; likely to cause death if left untreated).

Tumor marker: Substances that can be detected in higher than normal amounts in blood, urine, or body tissues with certain types of cancer; these may be produced by the tumor itself or the body's response to the tumor. Used with other tests and x-rays to detect and diagnose some types of cancers.

Ultrasound: Type of imaging technique using high-frequency sound waves; useful in diagnosis but not particularly accurate in assessment of tumor response.

White blood cells (WBC): Cells formed in the lymphatic system throughout the body and released in the circulating blood; important in fighting infection.

Wilms tumor: Cancerous tumor of the kidney usually found in children.

X-ray: Has a shorter wavelength than visible light. An x-ray machine uses ionizing electromagnetic radiation to bombard particles in a tight beam to a target area, causing the photons to reflect light in different intensities. A camera located behind the target area records the response of the target area in an image, where dense material like bone appears in white and soft tissues are grey to black.

Index